The Human Brain in Dissection

8.00

The Human Brain in Dissection

Second edition

DONALD G. MONTEMURRO, B.A., M.Sc., Ph.D.

Professor of Anatomy
The University of Western Ontario
London, Ontario, Canada

J. EDWARD BRUNI, B.Sc., M.Sc., Ph.D.

Associate Professor of Anatomy
The University of Manitoba
Winnipeg, Manitoba, Canada

New York · Oxford
OXFORD UNIVERSITY PRESS
1988

Oxford University Press

Oxford   New York   Toronto
Delhi   Bombay   Calcutta   Madras   Karachi
Petaling Jaya   Singapore   Hong Kong   Tokyo
Nairobi   Dar es Salaam   Cape Town
Melbourne   Auckland

and associated companies in
Beirut   Berlin   Ibadan   Nicosia

Published by Oxford University Press, Inc.,
200 Madison Avenue, New York, New York 10016

Oxford is a registered trademark of Oxford University Press

Library of Congress Cataloging-in-Publication Data
Montemurro, D. G. (Donald G.)
The human brain in dissection.
Bibliography: p.   Includes index.
1. Brain—Dissection. I. Bruni, J. Edward.
II. Title. [DNLM: 1. Brain—anatomy & histology.
2. Dissection. WL 300 M777h]
QM455.M68   1988   611′.81   87-24691
ISBN 0-19-504926-8

Printing (last digit): 9 8 7 6 5 4 3 2

Printed in the United States of America
on acid-free paper

TO OUR WIVES AND OUR CHILDREN: JUNE, MARIA, ANDREA

SONDRA, KIRSTEN, EDLYN, DAVID

Preface to the Second Edition

Many of our students over the past five years who have used this book in the neuroanatomy laboratory have stated verbally and in written comments that it is most helpful and easy to follow—don't change it! However, change is inevitable for its absence means stagnation.

We have corrected a few small errors in the labeling of some photographs. We have deleted some photographs that have not proven useful in the dissection exercise and have replaced them with ones more pertinent. We have inserted small photographs into some existing illustrations in order to amplify difficult anatomical points and into the Weigert-stained sections in order to illustrate the plane at which each of the sections was taken. We have deleted descriptive detail in some chapters that is of little significance to students of the health sciences. We have updated some of the textual material to conform to more modern knowledge of the structure and connections of the central nervous system.

A much more conspicuous change is the addition of an atlas of brain sections at the end of the book. Two major innovations in the diagnostic imaging of the brain, namely x-ray computerized tomography (C.T.) and magnetic resonance (M.R.) imagery, have changed the direction of anatomic teaching. Clinicians now view the living brain with remarkable clarity in two-dimensional planes with these techniques. It is essential that beginning students of the neurosciences become familiar with the appearance of both C.T. and M.R. images and be able to identify and locate the major neural structures seen in them. To this end, we have added 62 sections of the human brain cut in four different planes. Wherever possible we have included C.T. and M.R. images that correspond as closely as possible to the anatomic section. We are grateful to Dr. D. M. Pelz and Dr. A. J. Fox, both of the Departments of Diagnostic Radiology and Nuclear Medicine, and Clinical Neurological Sciences at the University of Western Ontario, who collaborated so readily with us in this endeavor. The C.T. and M.R. images are the result of their efforts.

In our experience, ten dissection periods each of two hours' duration are ideally required to complete the dissection exercise. If anatomic models and prosected specimens pertinent to the subject matter of each period are available in the laboratory, they can be helpful to both student and instructor. At the beginning of each period the students can be shown color videotapes twenty to forty minutes long (projected onto large screens) on the subject of the day's dissection. This allows the students to see what they should be able to identify and uncover in their own dissections. In this way very creditable dissections are often accomplished by beginning students. A series of these videotapes, based on the contents of this book, has been produced by the senior author and is available for purchase from Teaching Films Incorporated, Evanston, Illinois.

We realize that neuroanatomy syllabi may differ greatly from school to school depending upon the time available to teach the subject and the views of the instructors. Although the order of dissection recommended is roughly that shown in the Contents, we appreciate that this order may not be the one preferred by all instructors for a variety of reasons. If the order of presentation is to be altered we offer the following suggestions: the brain stem with attached cerebellum should be separated from the cerebrum by careful transection at the midbrain-diencephalic junction. Students should first examine and study the meninges (Chapter 4) and blood supply of the brain (Chapter 5) because the neural relationships of these structures will either be altered or destroyed during the course of subsequent dissection. Chapters 6 to 9 must be followed in the prescribed sequence to avoid missing structures, since the cerebrum is gradually dismembered in the process of the dissection.

We consider ourselves fortunate to have had the secretarial help of Mrs. Agnes Bentley, who typed the final draft of this manuscript.

London, Ontario   D. G. M.
Winnipeg, Manitoba   J. E. B.
July 1987

Contents

The Human Brain in Dissection

1

Introduction

The nervous system may be arbitrarily divided into two parts, the *peripheral nervous system* and the *central nervous system*. The peripheral nervous system is composed of 12 pairs of cranial nerves, 31 pairs of spinal nerves and their associated ganglia, and peripheral end organs. The central nervous system (CNS) consists of the *brain* and the *spinal cord*. These structures, which in the adult come to lie within the cavities of the skull and the vertebral column, respectively, derive from the midline ectoderm of the early embryo. A thickening and gradual infolding of this ectoderm forms the neural tube, which separates from and comes to lie beneath the superficial layer of ectoderm from which it derived. At an early stage of embryogenesis three primary swellings appear at the anterior end of this tube, which ultimately will form the brain of the adult; the remaining caudal portion of the tube ultimately forms the spinal cord. These primary swellings are called the *prosencephalon* (forebrain), the *mesencephalon* (midbrain), and the *rhombencephalon* (hindbrain).

By the fifth week of embryogenesis, the prosencephalon has divided into two entities, the *telencephalon* and the *diencephalon*. The telencephalon (endbrain) develops as two evaginations from the rostral prosencephalon, one on each side of the midline. These two telencephalic vesicles will eventually develop into the massive cerebral hemispheres of the adult. The original rostral limit of the neural tube is identified by the *lamina terminalis* in the adult. The caudal portion of the prosencephalon develops as the diencephalon (between brain), which in the adult consists of the *thalamus, hypothalamus, subthalamus,* and *epithalamus*. The mesencephalon remains undivided; in the adult brain the mesencephalon is also known as the *midbrain*. At the same time the forebrain is dividing, the rhombencephalon also divides into two secondary vesicles. The more anterior one is the *metencephalon* (after brain), which gives rise to the *pons* and the *cerebellum* of the adult. The more posterior one is the *myelencephalon* (marrow brain), which forms the *medulla oblongata* of the adult.

The cells of the nervous system are called *neurons*. The number is estimated to be about 100 billion. These cells are specialized for the reception of stimuli, the transduction of these stimuli into electrical impulses, and the conduction of these impulses to near or distant sites within the CNS. They also generate and conduct action potentials to muscles and glands, which result ultimately in motor and secretory activity. The nervous system is also composed of *neuroglial cells*, which subserve a variety of functions important to the integrity of the nervous system. These supporting cells are about ten times more numerous than neurons. Their number is estimated to be about one trillion, and they are reported to constitute half the volume of the brain.

Fixation of the CNS using the conventional formalin method results in an organ that has lost the soft gelatinous consistency of the living state. Fixed brains are firm and adopt a light straw or sand color. In many places the cell bodies of neurons are concentrated to form small or large aggregates of cells called *nuclei* or *ganglia*. In the fresh brain, these nuclei, because they contain few myelinated fibers, appear slightly darker in color than adjoining areas containing the

3

myelinated axons of these neurons. The term *gray matter* therefore has been applied traditionally to the former, the term *white matter* to the latter. Neither, however, is entirely gray nor white in the fixed brain specimen.

During the development of the brain, a bend occurs at the junction of the diencephalon and the midbrain. This is called the *mesencephalic flexure* and it is most evident in the brains of primates and man. As a result of this flexure, the cerebral hemispheres and diencephalon come to lie almost at a right angle to the long axis of the brain stem. This orientation occasionally leads to confusion in understanding the terminology employed to describe the adult human brain. It is advisable to become familiar with the following basic terms used in describing position, direction, and relationships in the CNS.

The term *superior* refers to structures at or directed toward the uppermost part of the cerebral hemispheres; *inferior* refers to structures in the opposite direction, i.e., toward the base of the cerebral hemispheres resting on the floor of the cranial cavity. *Rostral* (anterior) refers to structures directed toward the front or, as the name implies, toward the beak; *caudal* (posterior) refers to structures either located or directed in the opposite direction, toward the tail end. Within the brain stem, structures close to the back or posterior surface of the body are called *dorsal*, whereas structures close to the anterior surface are called *ventral*. Structures or fiber tracts that project to structures on the same side of the body are said to be *ipsilateral*, and those that are on or project to the opposite side of the body are said to be *contralateral*.

The *sagittal* (median) plane is a vertical plane of section passing through the sagittal suture of the skull and dividing the brain along its midline into two symmetrical halves. A *parasagittal* section of the brain is any vertical section on either side of the midline that parallels the sagittal suture and hence the long axis of the brain. *Medial* implies that a structure is located at or tends toward the median plane of the brain or spinal cord; *lateral implies the opposite*, i.e., away from the median plane or midline. A *coronal* (frontal) section is any vertical plane of section that parallels the coronal suture of the skull and is perpendicular to the median plane. This is the most common plane of brain section. A *horizontal* plane of section intersects both the coronal and median planes at right angles, thereby dividing the brain horizontally into upper and lower segments. The term *transverse* denotes planes of section placed crosswise or at a right angle to the long axis of a structure and is most appropriately applied with reference to the midbrain, pons, medulla, and spinal cord.

In dissection, as in any task, the choice and use of instruments imply some foreknowledge of what is to be accomplished. The artist chooses brushes by size and type to produce the desired visual effect on canvas; the cabinetmaker uses the tools appropriate to the design and finish to be produced in the wood. The choice of instruments will greatly affect the finished quality of the dissection described in the pages to follow. The only instruments required to effect a creditable dissection of the brain are a blunt probe, a scalpel, tissue forceps, scissors, a small spatula, and a brain knife. Long brain knives are usually provided by the institution.

The technique for dissection of the brain is different from that used for other parts of the body. It is performed mainly by blunt dissection with the handle end of the scalpel; the blade is seldom used. The objective is to disclose natural planes of cleavage produced by fiber bundles coursing in different directions in the interior of the brain. This is best achieved by pushing the blunt end of the scalpel handle into the substance of the brain and gently levering out a piece of brain tissue, allowing it to break away according to the manner in which it naturally separates (Fig. 1-1). The pieces so removed are usually fairly large, about one-half inch or larger in sizes. It will be appreciated that blunt dissection has major limitations; only large and quite discrete structures can be demonstrated in this way. In search of anything, it is an advantage to have some idea of what one is looking for. Students are well advised to identify the structure in question in one or more of the photographs provided before attempting to find it in their own brain specimens. This is most pertinent when dissecting the white matter of the hemisphere, for a knowledge of the location and direction of the structure will determine how the structure should be exposed. For example, the fibers of the external capsule appear to radiate from the limen insulae upward toward the superior longitudinal fasciculus (see Fig. 7-2). Therefore removing thin strips of white matter with a small flat spatula and tearing these strips upward with forceps or fingers in a radial manner will reveal the direction and arrangement of the fibers in this capsule. This technique is demonstrated in Figure 1-2. As with surgery on living tissue, it is essential that the field be kept clean and moist at all times. Be sure to dissect slowly and carefully until you are confident of the technique. Bon voyage.

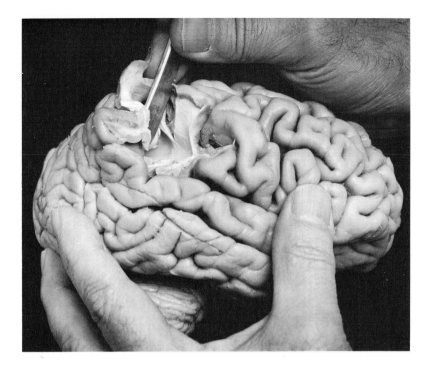

Figure 1-1. Technique for dissection of the brain. The blunt end of the scalpel is inserted into the cortex and a piece of tissue pried away so that it breaks along a natural cleavage plane.

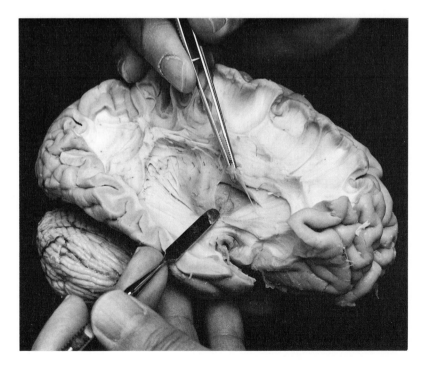

Figure 1-2. Technique for fine dissection of the white matter of the hemisphere using a small spatula and forceps.

5

2

Osteology of the Skull and Vertebral Column

The Skull

The *skull or cranium* is composed of 22 bones excluding the auditory ossicles. The bones of the skull with only a few exceptions (mandible, incus, malleus, and stapes) are immovable and united at joints called *sutures.* For descriptive purposes the bones of the skull can be further divided into *bones of the face* and *bones of the cranial cavity.* Examine the skull in lateral view, noting that an imaginary diagonal line extending from the upper margin of the orbit to the apex of the mastoid process approximately divides the facial bones of the skull from the bones of the cranial cavity (Fig. 2-1).

The *bones of the face* number 14 and include the mandible, vomer and paired lacrimal, nasal, palatine, zygomatic bones, and inferior nasal conchae. They contain and support the organs of special sensation, the oral and nasal passages, and provide attachment for the teeth and jaw. The *bones of the skull* that bound the cranial cavity and enclose the brain are 8 in number. They are the unpaired *frontal, ethmoid, sphenoid, and occipital bones and the paired temporal and parietal* bones.

The unpaired *frontal* bone forms the front and sides of the anterior part of the skull. The frontal bone articulates posteriorly with the paired *parietal* bones at the *coronal* suture, which extends from one temple to the other. The two parietal bones, which form the sides and posterior roof of the skull, are joined in the midline to form the *sagittal* suture. The sides of the skull are completed by the *temporal* and *sphenoid* bones. The posterior aspect of the skull is formed largely by the *occipital* bone, which articulates with the parietal bones at the *lambdoidal* suture. The flat bones forming the cranial cavity are pierced by small foramina (i.e., parietal, mastoid), which transmit *emissary veins* from the intracranial venous sinuses to superficial veins such as those in the scalp.

The union of these bones at their prominent sutures forms important craniometric landmarks and the basis for some commonly recognized neuronanatomical planes of section. The following points should now be identified on the surface of the skull with reference to Figure 2-1: The point at which the sagittal and coronal sutures meet is called the *bregma*. Note that the highest point on the circumference of the skull, called the *vertex,* is located on the sagittal suture about 3–4 cm behind the bregma. The point of junction of the sagittal and lambdoidal sutures is called the *lambda*. The point of junction of the frontal, sphenoid, parietal, and temporal bones on the lateral surface of the skull is called the *pterion*. It is of clinical significance because it is a thin region of the skull that directly overlies the anterior branch of the middle meningeal artery. The *asterion* is also located on the lateral surface of the skull at the point of junction of the parietal, temporal, and occipital bones.

The skull of the neonate differs in several important respects from

Figure 2-1. Lateral view of the skull showing the bones of the cranium and face and some craniometric points.

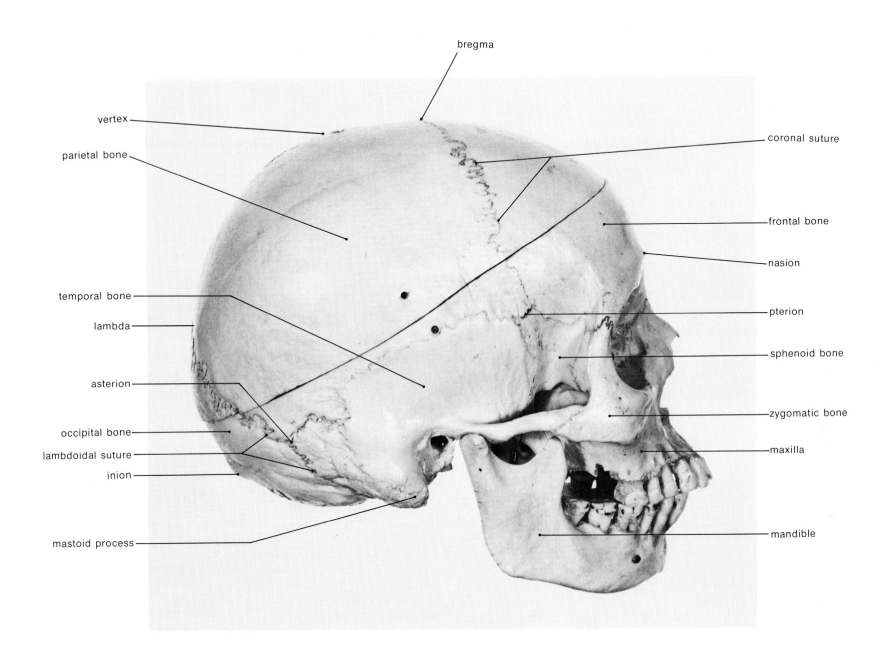

bregma

vertex

coronal suture

parietal bone

frontal bone

nasion

temporal bone

pterion

lambda

sphenoid bone

asterion

zygomatic bone

occipital bone

lambdoidal suture

maxilla

inion

mastoid process

mandible

the adult. Ossification is incomplete in the newborn and adjacent bones are not fused. In six locations the bones of the skull are separated by membrane-covered spaces called *fontanelles*. They are areas where the underlying brain is vulnerable to injury. The two larger and most regular fontanelles, the *anterior* and *posterior*, are of particular clinical interest. The largest is the diamond-shaped *anterior fontanelle* located in the midline at the junction of the coronal and sagittal sutures. It closes by approximation of adjacent bones within the second year of life. The *posterior fontanelle* is a triangular space located in the median plane posteriorly at the junction of the parietal and occipital bones. It usually closes at about 3 months after birth. The fontanelles are important because they provide ready access to venous sinus blood and to the cerebral ventricles as is sometimes required for investigative purposes. They may also be useful in early diagnosis of increased intracranial pressure.

The *calvaria* or *vault of the skull* roofs over the cranial cavity and its contents and is formed by the superior parts of the frontal, parietal, and occipital bones. Remove the calvaria from the specimen and examine the interior of the cranial cavity (Fig. 2-2). Note that its floor or base consists of three staired divisions called the *anterior*, *middle*, and *posterior cranial fossae*. The fossae are formed by the same bones (sphenoid, ethmoid, temporal, frontal, and occipital) that form the base of the skull. Note also that the fossae contain a number of openings called *foramina* through which pass all nerves and blood vessels to and from the brain. Identify on the specimen each of the following cranial fossae and their foramina referring to Figures 2-2 and 2-3.

Anterior Cranial Fossa

The anterior cranial fossa is the most rostral of the three bony compartments within the cranial cavity. Its anterior and lateral walls are formed by the inner surface of the *frontal bones*. In the midline, the floor of the fossa is formed anteriorly by the *cribriform plate* of the ethmoid bone and posteriorly by the *body of the sphenoid bone*. Most of the floor of the fossa is formed anterolaterally by the covex *orbital plates of the frontal bone;* posterolaterally it is bordered by a ridge of bone called the *lesser wing of the sphenoid bone*. Note the vertical midline projection from the ethmoid bone called the *crista galli* and the

median bony projection or *crest* of the frontal bone, which together provide attachment for the *falx cerebri* described in Chapter 4.

The anterior cranial fossa lodges the frontal lobes of the cerebral hemispheres and the surface of the orbital plates correspond closely with the pattern of orbital gyri and sulci on the undersurface of the frontal lobes. The lesser wings of the sphenoid bone lie in the interval between the frontal and temporal lobes known as the stem of the lateral sulcus and the anterior clinoid processes that arise medially from the lesser wings provide attachment for the anterior free margin of the tentorium cerebelli.

The olfactory bulbs lie on the cribriform plate on each side of the crista galli. Fascicles of nerve fibers called *fila olfactoria* originating from sensory receptor cells in the nasal mucosa enter the cranial cavity through the many foramina in the cribriform plate. Collectively these fila olfactoria form the olfactory nerve or cranial nerve I (CN I). Note the *foramen cecum* situated in the midline immediately in front of the crista galli. Through this opening an emissary vein passes from the nasal mucosa to the superior sagittal sinus.

Middle Cranial Fossa

The middle cranial fossa is the second of the three staired compartments. It is formed in the midline by the *body of the sphenoid* bone and laterally on each side by the *greater wings of the sphenoid* and *temporal* bones. The fossa is limited anteriorly by the lesser wing of the sphenoid bone and the sulcus chiasmaticus; posteriorly it is limited by the petrous temporal bone and dorsum sellae.

The middle cranial fossa accommodates the base of the diencephalon in the midline and the anterior part of the temporal lobes of the cerebral hemisphere in its laterally expanded region. The posterior part of the temporal lobes and the occipital lobes sit on a fold of dura mater called the tentorium cerebelli (Chapter 4), which roofs over the posterior cranial fossa. Now identify the following foramina in the floor of this fossa, which transmit important blood vessels and nerves:

Figure 2-2. The interior of the base of the skull showing the anterior, middle, and posterior cranial fossae and the foramina.

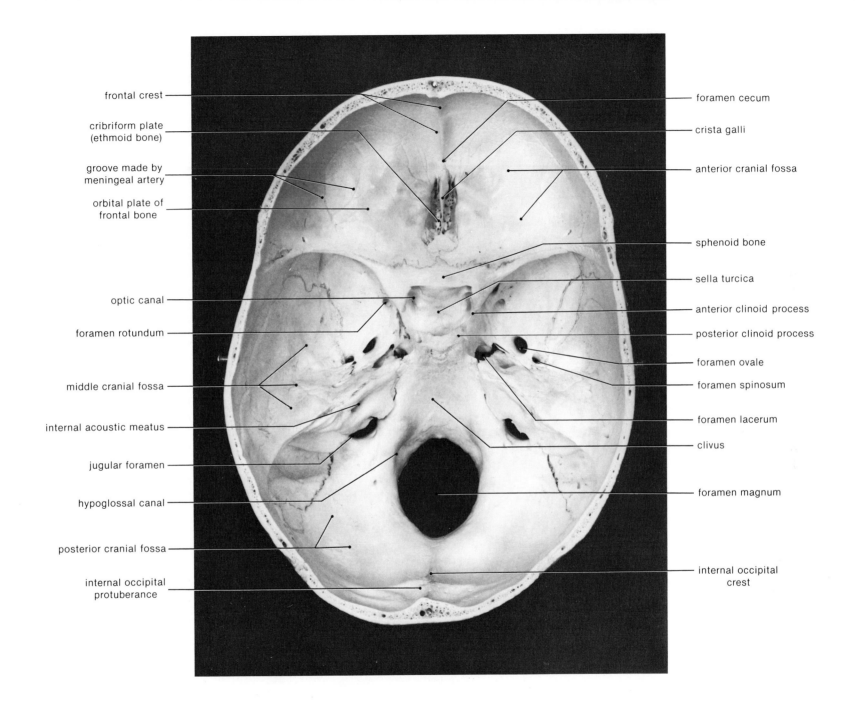

frontal crest

cribriform plate
(ethmoid bone)

groove made by
meningeal artery

orbital plate of
frontal bone

optic canal

foramen rotundum

middle cranial fossa

internal acoustic meatus

jugular foramen

hypoglossal canal

posterior cranial fossa

internal occipital
protuberance

foramen cecum

crista galli

anterior cranial fossa

sphenoid bone

sella turcica

anterior clinoid process

posterior clinoid process

foramen ovale

foramen spinosum

foramen lacerum

clivus

foramen magnum

internal occipital
crest

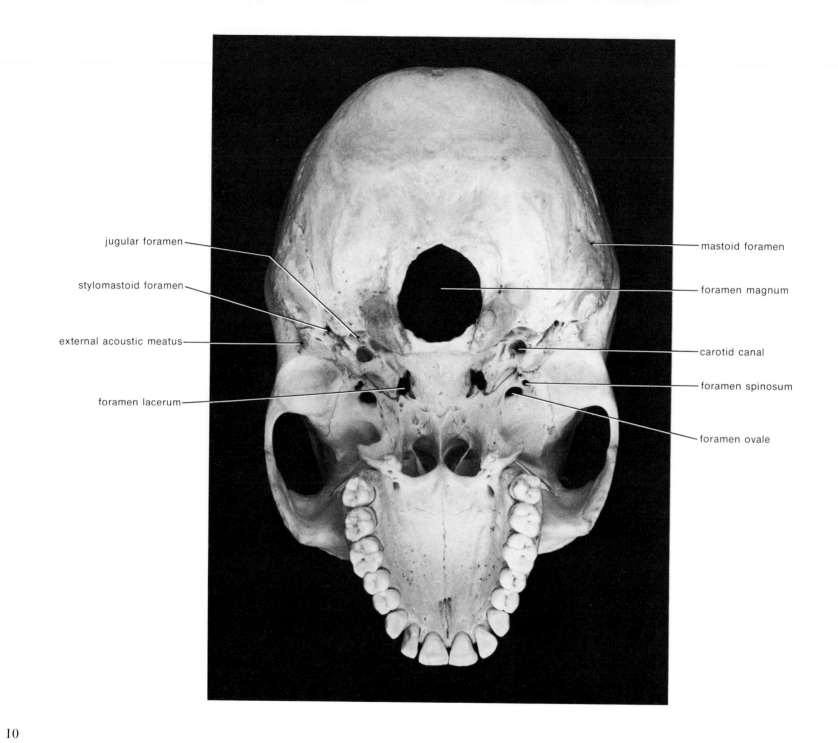

jugular foramen

stylomastoid foramen

external acoustic meatus

foramen lacerum

mastoid foramen

foramen magnum

carotid canal

foramen spinosum

foramen ovale

The *optic foramen (canal)* is an opening in the lesser wing of the sphenoid bone medial to the anterior clinoid process at each end of the sulcus chiasmaticus. The optic nerve (CN II) and the ophthalmic artery pass through this foramen to the orbital cavity.

The *superior orbital fissure* is located in the anterior wall of the middle fossa just lateral to the optic foramen. It is a narrow vertical opening between the greater and lesser wings of the sphenoid bone. It transmits the lacrimal, frontal, and nasociliary branches of the ophthalmic nerve (CN V_1), the oculomotor (CN III), the trochlear (CN IV), and the abducens (CN VI) nerves to the orbital cavity.

The *foramen rotundum* is a small round opening in the greater wing of the sphenoid bone below the superior orbital fissure. It conveys the maxillary branch (V_2) of the trigeminal nerve to the pterygopalatine fossa.

The *foramen ovale* is an oval opening in the greater wing of the sphenoid bone behind the foramen rotundum. It transmits the mandibular branch (V_3) of the trigeminal nerve to the infratemporal fossa. It also transmits the lesser petrosal nerve (a branch of CN IX) and the accessory meningeal artery. In addition it conveys an emissary vein from the cavernous sinus to the pterygoid venous plexus. These venous channels are of clinical significance because they represent potential routes by which infection can spread to the cranial cavity and its contents.

The *foramen spinosum* is a small opening immediately posterolateral to the foramen ovale. The meningeal branch of the mandibular nerve (V_3) and the middle meningeal artery enter the skull through this foramen. After entering the skull through the foramen the middle meningeal artery courses forward and laterally on the temporal bone and divides into a frontal or anterior and parietal or posterior branch. Their intracranial course can be traced by following the grooves left by them on the inner surface of the temporal, parietal, and frontal bones. The middle meningeal artery provides the blood supply to the dura mater and bone of the middle fossa and parietal areas. It is of particular clinical importance because of its susceptibility to rupture in the region of the temple (or pterion) where the overlying bone of the skull is thinnest. Rupture of this vessel can result in extradural hemorrhage, increased intracranial pressure, and death.

Figure 2-3. The exterior of the base of the skull.

The *foramen lacerum* is located medial to the foramen ovale between the greater wing of the sphenoid and the apex of the petrous temporal bones. The carotid canal, which contains the internal carotid artery, opens into the wall of the foramen lacerum. This artery enters the cranial cavity through the irregular opening of the foramen lacerum. The foramen also transmits the greater petrosal nerve which unites with the deep petrosal nerve to form the nerve of the pterygoid canal.

Posterior Cranial Fossa

The posterior cranial fossa is the largest and deepest of the three fossae. Anteromedially, it is bounded by the *body of the sphenoid bone* and the *clivus* of the occipital bone and anterolaterally by the *petrous temporal bone*. The floor and posterior wall of the fossa is formed by the *occipital bone;* the lateral walls are formed by the *occipital* bone and *mastoid part of the temporal bones*. A prominent vertical ridge of bone, the *internal occipital crest*, is located in the posterior midline of the fossa between two shallow depressions, the *cerebellar fossae*, which lodge the inferior hemispherical surface of the cerebellum.

The posterior fossa lodges the cerebellum, pons, and medulla oblongata. The tentorium cerebelli extends forward from the occipital bone to the pertous temporal bone and separates the posterior fossa below from the occipital and posterior temporal lobes of the cerebral hemispheres above. The vertical dural fold, the falx cerebelli, is attached to the internal occipital crest. As with the other two fossae, the posterior cranial fossa contains several foramina of importance that should now be identified.

The largest and most conspicuous is the central opening in the floor of the fossa called the *foramen magnum*. The medulla oblongata continues through this foramen as the cervical cord. The spinal root of the accessory nerve (CN XI) and the paired vertebral arteries ascend into the cranial cavity through the foramen magnum. In addition the anterior and posterior spinal arteries also descend through this foramen.

The *hypoglossal canal* is a small opening located on the anterolateral wall of the posterior fossa just above the margin of the foramen magnum. It conducts the hypoglossal nerve (CN XII) from the cranial cavity.

The *internal acoustic* (or *auditory*) *meatus* is a small opening on the

Table 2-1. Foramina at the Base of the Skull and the Structures They Transmit

Foramina	Contents
Anterior Cranial Fossa	
Foramen cecum	Emissary vein from nasal mucosa to superior sagittal sinus
Foramina of cribriform plate	Olfactory nerves (CN I)
Middle Cranial Fossa	
Optic foramen	Optic nerve (CN II)
	Ophthalmic artery
Superior orbital fissure	Oculomotor nerve (CN III)
	Trochlear nerve (CN IV)
	Ophthalmic nerve (branch of V_1)
	Abducens nerve (CN VI)
Foramen rotundum	Maxillary nerve (CN V_2)
Foramen ovale	Mandibular nerve (CN V_3)
	Lesser petrosal nerve
	Accessory meningeal artery
	Emissary veins
Foramen spinosum	Middle meningeal artery
	Meningeal nerve (CN V_3)
Foramen lacerum	Internal carotid artery
	Greater petrosal nerve
Posterior Cranial Fossa	
Internal auditory meatus	Facial nerve (CN VII)
	Vestibulocochlear nerve (CN VIII)
	Labyrinthine artery and vein
Jugular foramen	Inferior petrosal sinus
	Glossopharyngeal nerve (CN IX)
	Vagus nerve (CN X)
	Accessory nerve (CN XI)
	Sigmoid sinus
Hypoglossal canal	Hypoglossal nerve (CN XII)
Foramen magnum	Medulla oblongata/spinal cord
	Accessory nerve (CN XI) spinal root
	Vertebral arteries
	Anterior and posterior spinal arteries
	Internal vertebral venous plexus communicating with occipital and basilar sinuses

anterolateral wall of the posterior fossa, which conveys the facial nerve (CN VII), vestibulocochlear (CN VIII), and labyrinthine vessels to the inner ear.

Below the internal acoustic meatus is a large irregular opening between the petrous temporal and occipital bones called the *jugular foramen*. It transmits the accessory (CN XI), vagus (CN X), and glossopharyngeal (CN IX) nerves. In addition the inferior petrosal and sigmoid sinuses pass through the foramen to enter the internal jugular vein.

With the assistance of the summary table (Table 2-1) review the foramina located at the base of the skull and their contents.

The Vertebral Column

The vertebral column consists of 33 separate bones or *vertebrae* stacked on top of each other to form a continuous structure measuring approximately 72–75 cm in length. The vertebrae separated by fibrocartilaginous intervertebral disks are united at articular processes and are held firmly together by ligaments. The vertebral column supports the head and trunk and houses and protects the spinal cord.

The vertebral column is divided into 5 regions: *cervical, thoracic, lumbar, sacral,* and *coccygeal*. There are 7 cervical, 12 thoracic, and 5 lumbar vertebrae. Together these comprise the 24 true or presacral vertebrae. The 5 sacral vertebrae and the 4 coccygeal vertebrae are fused together to form 2 large composite vertebrae, the sacrum and the coccyx.

Although vertebrae exhibit some unique regional characteristics, they do possess a common basic structure. All vertebrae are composed of an anteriorly located *body* or *centrum* and a posterior *neural or vertebral arch* (Fig. 2-4). The centrum is a large cylindrical structure, which serves principally a weight-bearing function. The bodies of adjoining vertebrae are separated by fibrocartilagenous *intervertebral disks* and are united by anterior and posterior ligaments. Each neural arch is formed by two pedicles, two laminae, and various projecting bony processes (transverse, spinous, and articular processes). The *pedicles* are short stout processes, which project posteri-

Figure 2-4. Four thoracic vertebrae viewed from above and from the side showing their typical structure.

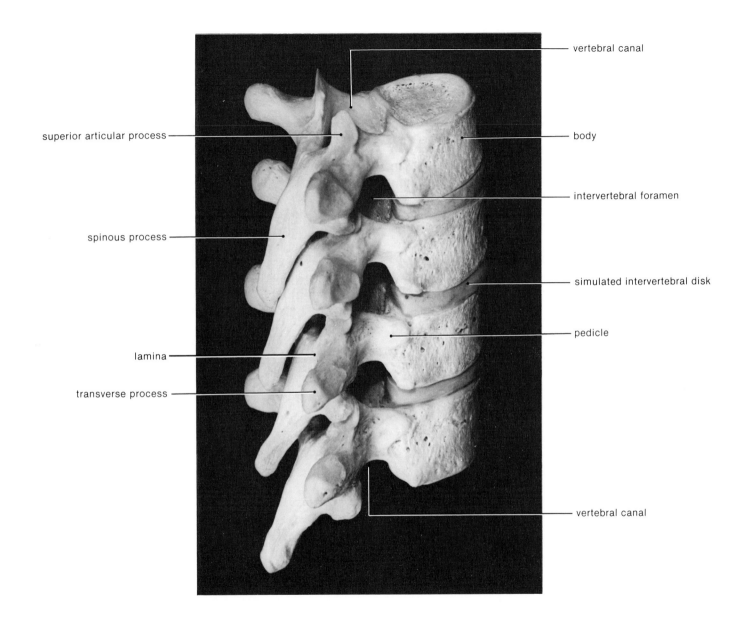

vertebral canal

superior articular process

body

intervertebral foramen

spinous process

simulated intervertebral disk

pedicle

lamina

transverse process

vertebral canal

orly from the posterolateral surface of the body of the vertebrae. The pedicles are notched on their upper and lower surfaces and the apposition of these notches from pedicles of contiguous vertebrae form the *intervertebral foramina* through which spinal nerves pass. The broad flat *laminae* extend from the pedicles and unite in the postèrior midline. Two transverse processes and two superior and two inferior articular processes arise at the junction of the pedicles and laminae. A single *spinous process* emerges from the point of union of the two laminae in the posterior midline. The transverse and spinous processes provide for the attachment of muscles and ligaments. Unlike cervical and thoracic vertebrae the laminae of lumbar vertebrae do not overlap and the spinous processes are not directed obliquely downward and backward. This readily allows the insertion of a needle into the intervertebral space between the spinous processes as required in lumbar puncture (Chapter 12).

The centrum and neural arch of each vertebra together enclose a *vertebral foramen*. Superimposition of these foramina forms the *vertebral canal*, which houses and protects the spinal cord. The size and shape of the vertebral canal vary regionally. In order to accommodate the large size of the cervical spinal cord, the vertebral foramen in the cervical region is large and triangular in outline. At thoracic levels the vertebral foramen is smaller than other levels and circular in shape. The vertebral foramen is oval in outline at lumbar levels and larger than thoracic but smaller in size than at cervical levels.

There are usually five rudimentary sacral vertebrae, which are fused together to form a single bone, the *sacrum*. The sacrum encloses a flattened triangular vertebral canal that contains the cauda equina and filum terminale. The concave pelvic surface of the sacrum has four large anterior sacral foramina through which the ventral or anterior rami of the first four sacral nerves emerge. The posterior or dorsal rami of the first four sacral nerves exit via the dorsal sacral foramina on posterior surface of the sacrum. The laminae of the fifth and sometimes fourth sacral segments fail to fuse in the posterior midline producing an opening to the vertebral canal, the *sacral hiatus*. Through this opening the filum terminale, fifth sacral, and coccygeal spinal nerve roots emerge. The apex of the sacrum articulates with the *coccyx* which consists of the remains of the bodies of four vertebrae fused to form a single small triangular bone. The location of spinal cord segments relative to their bony vertebral investment is important clinically and is described in Chapter 12.

3

General Structure of the Brain

At birth, the human brain weighs approximately 300–400 g, and its volume is only one-fourth that of the adult brain. By the end of the first year, the brain increases in weight to approximately 800–1000 g and attains 75% of its adult volume. This is attributable to the growth of neurons, neuroglial cells, cerebral blood vessels, and particularly the myelination of axons. By late childhood the brain attains its full adult weight of approximately 1400 g (range 1200–1700 g), which represents only about 2% of the adult body weight. The brain of the female is said to weigh less (100 g) than that of the male; however, in proportion to body weight these differences are negligible. Within normal limits—that is, in the absence of overt pathology—there is no evidence to correlate the size or weight of the brain with ability or intelligence. These faculties are more appropriately related to the microscopic and biochemical organization of neural tissue in some yet ill-defined way than they are to the gross morphology, size, or weight of the brain.

A cursory survey of the main features of the brain is necessary for orientation before it is studied in detail. Place the brain specimen with its right side resting on the table or tray. Most of the brain seen from this view is the left *cerebral hemisphere* (see Fig. 6-2). Both the left and the right cerebral hemispheres are composed of a superficial layer of gray matter, the *cerebral cortex,* a core of *subcortical white matter,* and a group of large nuclei within the depths of each hemisphere that are known collectively as the *telencephalic* or *basal ganglia.* Recall that the cerebral hemispheres are formed by massive growth of the telencephalon in the embryo. The cortex is made up of a layer of gray matter that is thrown into many convolutions and depressions, the result of which is to greatly increase its surface area within the confined space of the cranium. The total surface area of the cortex is estimated to be 285,000 mm^2, (about 3 ft^2) and the cortex is said to contain as many as 14 billion neurons.

The thickness of the surface layer of gray matter varies from place to place, the average thickness being about 2.5 mm; however, it is usually thicker at the apices of the convolutions than it is in the depths of the depressions. It is thickest in the region of the motor cortex of the precentral gyrus (4.5 mm) and thinnest in the visual cortex of the occipital lobe (1.5 mm). The subcortical white matter is composed of vast numbers of fibers that interconnect various cortical areas and project to and from the brain stem and spinal cord. The *corpus striatum* is a group of large nuclei located near the base of the hemisphere, which subserves a motor function.

Situated beneath the posterior portion of the two hemispheres is the *cerebellum,* which is readily identified by the many long slender convolutions on its surface. These convolutions are known as *cerebellar folia* (Fig. 3-1, Fig. 6-2). Like the cerebral hemispheres, the cerebellum consists of a thin layer of superficial gray matter, the *cerebellar cortex,* and a central core of subcortical white matter in which are embedded a group of deep cerebellar nuclei (Figs. 13-1, 13-23, and 13-41). The cerebellum is concerned largely but not exclusively with maintenance of equilibrium and synergism of muscle action.

Turn the brain so that the inferior surface is now toward you. Most of the surface thus presented is again that of the cerebral hemispheres. The ventral surface of the cerebellum is also evident. Now direct your attention to the structures in the midline. Beginning at the anterior end, notice the oval *olfactory bulb* and the elongated *olfactory tract* attached to it (Fig. 3-1). These structures form part of the *rhinencephalon*, or nose brain. Continuing posteriorly, the cut ends of the *optic nerves* are visible. They converge in the midline to form the *optic chiasma* and then diverge as the *optic tracts*. These represent part of the visual apparatus of the brain. Just behind the optic chiasma, notice two small eminences near the midline. These are the *mamillary bodies* of the hypothalamus. The neural tissue located between the optic chiasma and the mamillary bodies (including the mamillary bodies) is the only portion of the *diencephalon* visible on the exterior of the brain. Behind and lateral to the mamillary bodies, notice a robust column of white matter on each side. These corrugated columns converging toward the pons form part of the *cerebral peduncles* of the midbrain. They convey fibers projecting from many regions of the cerebral cortex to the brain stem and spinal cord. The remainder of the midbrain cannot be seen at this stage; it will be examined later in Chapter 10.

The next short segment of the brain stem is the *pons*. Notice the single *basilar artery* lying in a shallow groove in the midline of the pons (see Fig. 5-1 and Fig. 13-1). The ventral part of the pons is a stout bridge of gray and white matter consisting of transversely oriented fibers that project to the cerebellum and form the *middle cerebellar peduncles*. Notice the large cranial nerve root attached to the ventrolateral surface of the pons. This is the fifth cranial nerve, the *trigeminal nerve*. The remainder of the brain stem is the *medulla oblongata*. The deep groove running longitudinally in the midline of the medulla is the *ventral median fissure*, which is continuous with the same fissure on the ventral surface of the spinal cord (Figs. 3-1 and 12-2). The longitudinal ridges lying one on each side of this fissure are the *pyramids*, formed by the fibers of the *corticospinal tracts*. These fibers originate in various regions of the cerebral cortex and ultimately terminate at successive levels of the spinal cord. They are responsible in part for the execution of volitional movements and are components of the *pyramidal motor system*. Notice a prominent swelling, the *olive*, on each lateral surface of the medulla. The olive marks the position of a large nucleus, the *inferior olivary nucleus*, which is associated with the cerebellum (see Fig. 13-21).

Emerging from the medulla, notice several fine filaments ar-ranged in longitudinal rows; these are rootlets of cranial nerves and will be examined in detail in Chapter 10. The medulla, pons, and midbrain are known collectively as the *brain stem*. Besides containing nuclei of the cranial nerves, the brain stem contains many other nuclei and the ascending and descending fiber tracts to and from the cerebral cortex, diencephalon, cerebellum, and spinal cord.

The spinal cord is the caudal continuation of the medulla. In the 3-month-old fetus the spinal cord is the same length as the vertebral column. The rate of growth of the vertebral column subsequently outstrips that of the spinal cord, however, so that at birth the cord ends at the level of the third lumbar vertebra. In the adult the cord is only about 45 cm long and does not extend the full length of the vertebral column. It occupies only the upper two-thirds of the vertebral canal, ending at the level between the first and the second lumbar vertebra.

The spinal cord is a continuous cylinder of gray and white matter (Fig. 12-1). Unlike the cerebral cortex, the gray matter occupies the central core of the cylinder, whereas the ascending and descending fiber tracts constituting the white matter are located peripherally. In transverse section the gray matter of the spinal cord, which consists of cell columns, has roughly the shape of the letter H, formed by two *dorsal* (posterior) *horns* and two *ventral* (anterior) *horns* of gray matter joined in the middle (Fig. 12-3). The spinal cord is a continuum, although it may appear segmented because of the emergence of spinal nerves along its lateral margin. There are 31 pairs of spinal nerves: 8 cervical, 12 thoracic, 5 lumbar, 5 sacral, and 1 coccygeal. The roots of these nerves that enter the spinal cord on its dorsolateral surface are sensory in function, whereas those that emerge from the ventrolateral surface are motor in function (Fig. 12-2). A more complete description of the spinal cord is provided in Chapter 12.

Figure 3-1. View of the inferior surface of the brain showing some of the more prominent features of the cerebral hemispheres, diencephalon, midbrain, pons, medulla oblongata, and cerebellum.

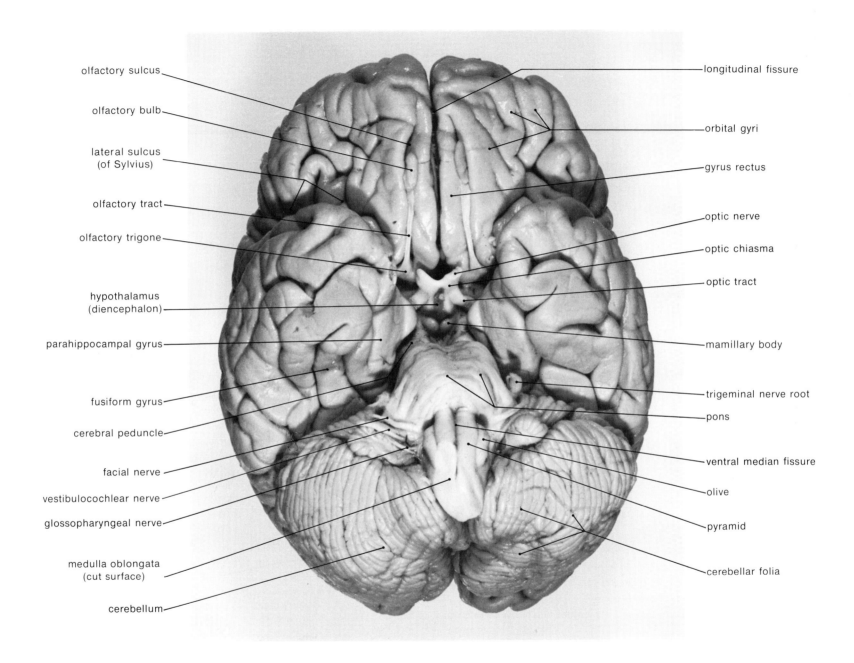

olfactory sulcus

olfactory bulb

lateral sulcus
(of Sylvius)

olfactory tract

olfactory trigone

hypothalamus
(diencephalon)

parahippocampal gyrus

fusiform gyrus

cerebral peduncle

facial nerve

vestibulocochlear nerve

glossopharyngeal nerve

medulla oblongata
(cut surface)

cerebellum

longitudinal fissure

orbital gyri

gyrus rectus

optic nerve

optic chiasma

optic tract

mamillary body

trigeminal nerve root

pons

ventral median fissure

olive

pyramid

cerebellar folia

17

4

Meninges

Few brain specimens obtained from hospital pathology departments are invested with complete meningeal coverings. Therefore, one or two demonstration specimens complete with dura mater should be provided for this laboratory. These specimens should be dissected in such a way as to expose the several dural septa and the dural venous sinuses. Suitable models may be employed in lieu of demonstration specimens. The brain specimen that you have been provided with will be used for all subsequent dissections; it should be handled carefully and with respect.

The brain and spinal cord are enveloped by three membranous layers called the *meninges*. The outer layer is the *dura mater,* or *pachymeninx,* and the inner layer is the *pia mater;* the *arachnoid* is located between the two. The pia mater and the arachnoid are referred to collectively as the *leptomeninges.*

Dura Mater

The *cranial dura* probably will not be present on many specimens, but on a few there may be an incomplete cap of dura covering the superior surface of the brain. Feel the tough texture of the dura and recall its histologic structure. The dura enveloping the brain is composed of two layers of dense fibrous connective tissue. The outer or *endosteal layer* is adherent to the inner surface of the cranial bones and serves as the periosteum. Some authors therefore prefer to call this the *periosteal layer.* The *meningeal layer* forms the inner cerebral layer of this tough connective tissue covering. It should be emphasized that except for a few locations within the cranial cavity where the two layers are separated, they are closely apposed and indistin-

guishable from one another. The dura surrounding the spinal cord differs from the cranial dura. The spinal dura is continuous with only the meningeal layer of the cranial dura. The outer or endosteal layer here is represented by the periosteum of the vertebrae, which is separated from the spinal dura by a space containing adipose and areolar tissue. This space is called the *epidural space.* Advantage is taken of this space in clinical medicine for the introduction of local anesthetic agents. A more detailed description of the dural and leptomeningeal investments of the spinal cord is provided in Chapter 12.

At four locations the meningeal layer of the cranial dura mater is reflected inward to form *dural reflections* or *septa* that incompletely divide the cranial cavity into compartments. With the aid of demonstration specimens or models, and the photographs provided in Figure 4-1, identify the following important dural reflections:

1. The *falx cerebri* is a sickle-shaped vertical septum located in the

---

Figure 4-1. Dissection of the left half of the head and brain to show the relationship of the dural septa (falx cerebri and tentorium cerebelli) with the dural venous sinuses. The sinuses have been filled with colored wax. The three small photographs are interior views of the base of the skull into which have been fitted replicas of the dural septa and dural venous sinuses: (a) The diaphragma sellae and the cavernous sinus forming the roof of the sella turcica. The falx cerebelli and occipital sinus attached to the internal occipital crest. (b) The tentorium cerebelli with the transverse sinuses and superior petrosal sinuses at its attached margin and the straight sinus in the midline has been added. (c) The falx cerebri with its superior sagittal sinus at the attached margin and the inferior sagittal sinus at the free margin have been added.

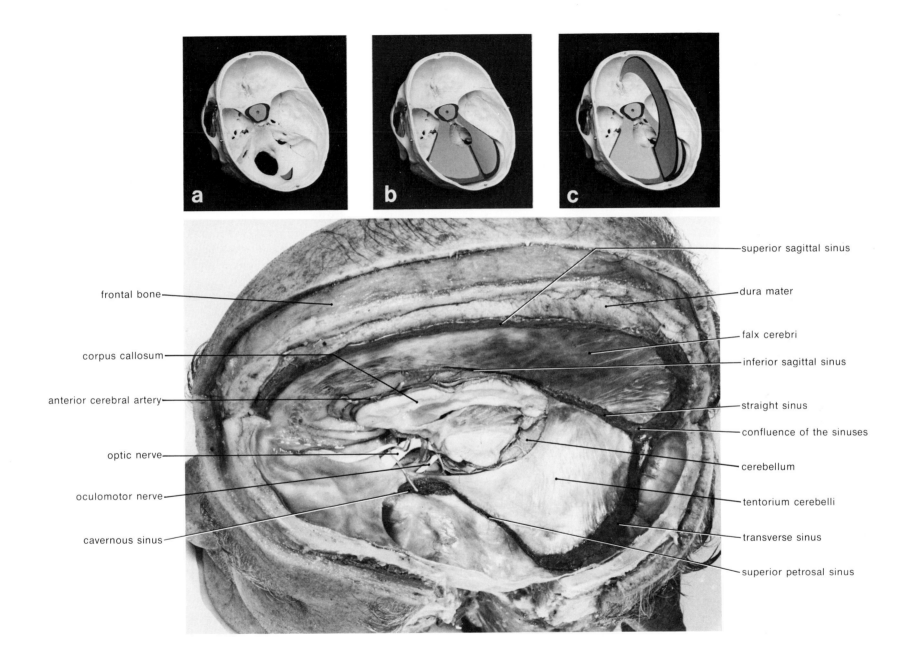

superior sagittal sinus

frontal bone

dura mater

falx cerebri

corpus callosum

inferior sagittal sinus

anterior cerebral artery

straight sinus

confluence of the sinuses

optic nerve

cerebellum

oculomotor nerve

tentorium cerebelli

transverse sinus

cavernous sinus

superior petrosal sinus

19

longitudinal fissure between the two cerebral hemispheres (Fig. 4-1). It extends from the *crista galli* of the ethmoid bone to the *internal occipital protuberance* and is attached to the midline of the upper surface of the tentorium cerebelli.

2. The *tentorium cerebelli* extends horizontally between the occipital lobes of the cerebrum above and the cerebellum below. Its attachment to the falx along the median plane gives the tentorium a tent-like configuration. Its peripheral border is attached to the occipital and parietal bones and to the petrous portion of the temporal bones. Its central border is free and forms a large horseshoe-shaped opening occupied by the midbrain and the superior cerebellar vermis. This opening is known as the *tentorial incisure* or *notch*. The anterior ends of the free and attached margins of the tentorium are fixed to the *anterior* and *posterior clinoid processes,* respectively (Fig. 2-2; see also Fig. 4-1b and 4-1c). The tentorium cerebelli forms a thick dural roof over the posterior cranial fossa.

3. The *falx cerebelli* is a small vertical midline septum located below the tentorium cerebelli. It is attached to the inferior surface of the tentorium above and to the internal occipital crest posteriorly. It projects into the *posterior cerebellar incisure,* which partially separates the hemispheres of the cerebellum (Fig. 4-1a).

4. The *diaphragma sellae* is a horizontal reflection of dura located ventral to the brain that roofs over the sella turcica. It is perforated centrally by the *hypophysial stalk,* which connects the pituitary gland (hypophysis cerebri) to the brain (Fig. 4-1a–c).

Not only does the dura mater provide protection and support for the brain, but the main septa dividing the cranial cavity into compartments restrict the movement of the brain *in situ.* This structural arrangement may be considered an additional means of protection for the brain against sudden and violent movement of the head.

Dural Venous Sinuses

At certain locations, usually the free and fixed margins of dural septa, and outer and inner layers of the dura are separated to form endothelial-lined channels. These channels provide for the venous drainage of blood from the brain and are called the *dural venous sinuses.* The sinuses communicate with meningeal veins and the *diploic* veins of the cranial bones, as well as with the veins of the scalp via *emissary* veins. Although the arterial blood supply and the venous drainage of the brain are examined in Chapter 5, it is profitable to examine the venous sinuses at this stage of the dissection.

Unless provided with a brain specimen complete with dural investment, you will have to identify the following venous sinuses using demonstration specimens and models.

1. The *superior sagittal sinus* is situated in the sagittal plane within the attached borders of the falx cerebri (Fig. 4-1 and 4-1c). It originates at the level of the foramen cecum and enlarges as it passes backward to the internal occipital protuberance. It deviates to one side, usually to the right, at the internal occipital protuberance and continues as the right *transverse sinus.* With the blade of the scalpel or with sharp scissors incise the sinus in the midline for a distance of 4–6 cm about midway between the frontal and occipital poles of the hemisphere. Retract the cut edges or remove the dural roof of the sinus by careful dissection with forceps and scalpel blade. Note that the sinus is roughly triangular in shape, that it receives the superior cerebral veins, and that it communicates with large *venous lacunae* along its lateral borders (Fig. 4-2). These lacunae contain protrusions from the underlying arachnoid, which are called *arachnoid villi.* Accumulations of enlarged arachnoid villi form macroscopically visible *arachnoid granulations (Pacchionian bodies),* which often become calcified with age. Arachnoid villi are the major site of passage of cerebrospinal fluid from the subarachnoid space into the general systemic circulation. The superior sagittal sinus also receives veins from the meninges, diploe, scalp, and nose. These channels of communication are important clinically because they provide the anatomic route by which infection may spread to the cranial cavity and brain.

2. The *inferior sagittal sinus* is smaller than the superior and occupies the inferior free border of the falx cerebri (Fig. 4-1 and 4-1c). At its posterior limit it is joined by the *great cerebral vein (of Galen)* to form the *straight sinus (sinus rectus).*

3. The *straight sinus,* after receiving the inferior sagittal sinus and

Figure 4-2. The superior sagittal sinus and the lateral venous lacunae. The dural roof of the sinus and the lacunae has been removed to show the arachnoid granulations. The dark threads are inserted in the points of communication between the sinus and the venous lacunae.

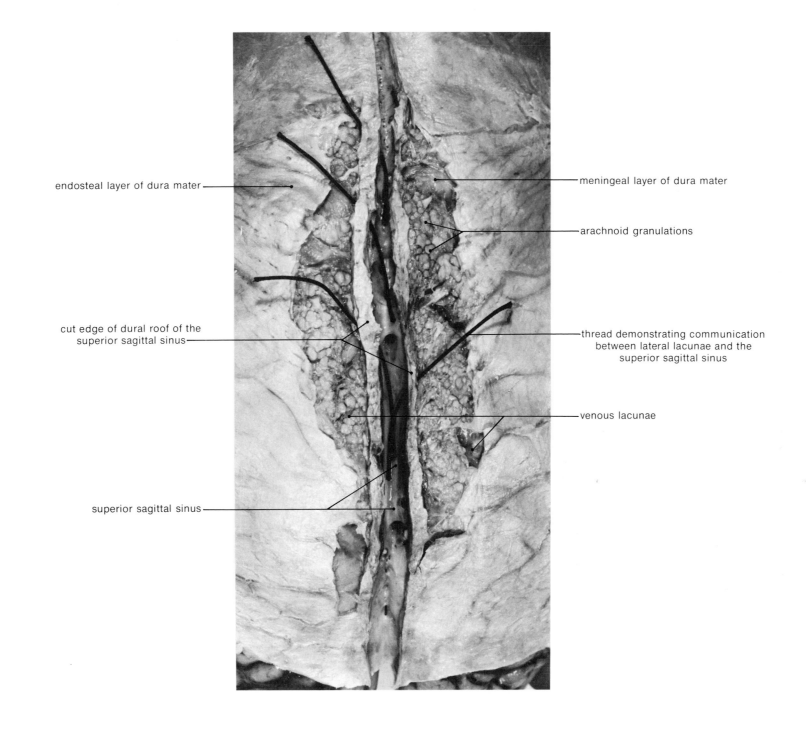

endosteal layer of dura mater

meningeal layer of dura mater

arachnoid granulations

cut edge of dural roof of the superior sagittal sinus

thread demonstrating communication between lateral lacunae and the superior sagittal sinus

venous lacunae

superior sagittal sinus

the great cerebral vein, extends caudally along the midline attachment of the falx cerebri to the superior surface of the tentorium cerebelli (Fig. 4-1, 4-1b, and 4-1c). The straight sinus empties into the transverse sinus, usually the left transverse sinus. The junction of the great cerebral vein with the straight sinus is of clinical importance because obstruction of the vein in this location may occur as the result of space-occupying lesions that alter the normal anatomic relationship between the tentorium and the midbrain. Obstruction of outflow from the great cerebral vein affects the production of cerebrospinal fluid by the choroid plexuses.

4. The two *transverse sinuses* pass from the internal occipital protuberance anterolaterally along the fixed margin of the tentorium cerebelli to the occipital and parietal bones (Fig. 4-1, 4-1b, and 4-1c). At the point of junction of the parietal, temporal, and occipital bones (the asterion) the transverse sinuses curve abruptly downward and medially. At this point they receive the *superior petrosal sinuses* and continue as the *sigmoid sinuses*. The two sigmoid sinuses curve downward and medially to empty into the *internal jugular veins* within the jugular foramen.

The *confluence of the sinuses* refers to a dilatation of the venous channel at the level of the internal occipital protuberance, where the superior sagittal sinus, straight sinus, occipital sinus, and two transverse sinuses converge.

5. The *cavernous sinuses* are an irregular plexiform network of venous channels on each side of the body of the sphenoid bone extending from the superior orbital fissure to the apex of the petrous temporal bone (Fig. 4-1a). Venous channels located in the attached anterior and posterior margins of the diaphragma sellae interconnect the cavernous sinus of each side. These *intercavernous sinuses*, along with the two cavernous sinuses, are sometimes referred to as the *circular sinus*. Anterolaterally, the cavernous sinuses receive the two *sphenoparietal sinuses*, which lie along the lesser wing of the sphenoid bone. The superficial, middle, and inferior cerebral veins and the ophthalmic veins also open into the cavernous sinus. The internal carotid artery and the abducens nerve (CN VI) pass through the cavernous sinus and are therefore vulnerable in their course to thrombosis of the sinus. The oculomotor (CN III) and trochlear nerves (CN IV) and the ophthalmic (V$_1$) and maxillary (V$_2$) divisions of the trigeminal nerve (CN V) pass forward within the lateral wall of the cavernous sinus. The cavernous sinus is important clinically because

it communicates with veins from the face, nose, and pharynx providing a route by which infections in these areas may spread to the cavernous sinus. Because of its contents, infections that lead to thrombosis of this sinus can have widespread neurologic consequences.

The cavernous sinuses drain posteriorly into the transverse sinuses and the internal jugular veins via two smaller sinuses, the superior and the inferior petrosal sinuses, respectively. The *superior petrosal* sinus is situated within the margins of the tentorium attached to the petrous portion of the temporal bone. The *inferior petrosal* sinus runs along a groove between the petrous temporal and occipital bones to the jugular foramen. A *basilar plexus* of venous channels situated on the clivus interconnects the two inferior petrosal sinuses and communicates with the anterior internal vertebral venous plexus.

6. The posterior margin of the falx cerebelli attached to the internal occipital crest encloses the small vertically oriented *occipital sinus*, which drains into the confluence of the sinuses (Fig. 4-1a). It communicates with the internal venous plexus of the vertebral canal.

Arachnoid Mater

The *arachnoid* mater is a delicate membrane that does not follow the contour of the brain, but rather is closely adherent to the inner layer of the dura mater being separated from it by a narrow *subdural space*. This space, which contains a thin film of fluid, is in reality more of a potential space than a real one. The interval between the arachnoid and the innermost meningeal layer, the pia mater, is the *subarachnoid space*. This space contains cerebrospinal fluid and is bridged by connective tissue trabeculae that attach the arachnoid to the pia mater. The trabeculae are visible to the unaided eye particularly in some locations such as the *subarachnoid cisterns* where the size of the subarachnoid space is greatly enlarged. At autopsy when the brain is removed, cerebrospinal fluid escapes and the arachnoid collapses onto the pia mater. The thin transparent connective tissue membrane that is seen investing the brain specimen is therefore the arachnoid (Figs. 4-3 and 5-3). The pia mater cannot be easily iden-

Figure 4-3. Posterior view of the brain showing the location of the cisterna magna in the subarachnoid space between the medulla oblongata and the cerebellum.

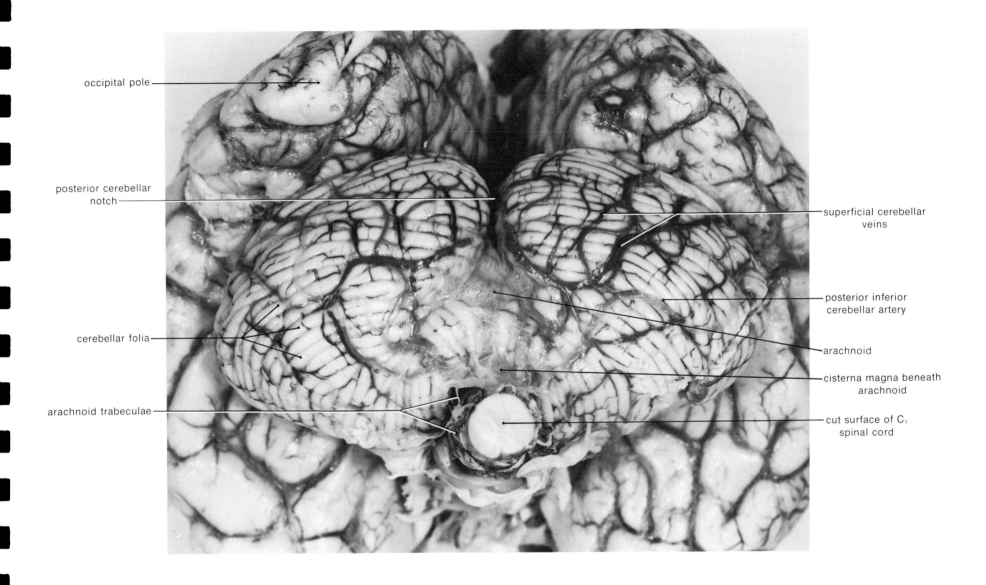

occipital pole

posterior cerebellar notch

superficial cerebellar veins

posterior inferior cerebellar artery

cerebellar folia

arachnoid

cisterna magna beneath arachnoid

arachnoid trabeculae

cut surface of C₁ spinal cord

tified. Incise a short length of arachnoid overlying a sulcus of the brain and notice that the blood vessels of the brain are wholly contained within the subarachnoid space.

Subarachnoid Cisterns

Because the arachnoid follows the contour of the dura while the pia is closely adherent to the convoluted surface of the brain, the two components of the leptomeninges are found to be widely separated in certain locations. The resulting enlarged subarachnoid space forms a number of freely communicating *subarachnoid cisterns*. The location of the major cisterns surrounding the brain are shown in Figure 4-4. The following cisterns should be identified in your brain specimen at this stage:

1. The *cerebellomedullary cistern (cisterna magna)* is located in the angle formed by the dorsal surface of the medulla oblongata and the inferior surface of the cerebellum (Fig. 4-3). It is one of the largest of the cisterns. Make a midline incision in the arachnoid forming the roof of this cistern. Now separate the cerebellum and the medulla by gently exerting a little downward pressure on the medulla. Notice the irregular opening into the cavity thus exposed. The cavity is the *fourth ventricle;* the opening is the *median aperture of the fourth ventricle (foramen of Magendie),* through which cerebrospinal fluid, formed within the ventricles, reaches the subarachnoid space. Note also the choroid plexus suspended from the roof of the fourth ventricle. Turn the brain over so that the ventral (inferior) surface is now toward you.

2. The *pontine cistern* is an extensive space enclosing the ventral surface of the pons. Locate the angle formed by the junction of the pons with the cerebellum and the medulla. A small tuft of choroid plexus protruding from the right and left sides marks the location of the *lateral apertures of the fourth ventricle (foramina of Luschka).* Cerebrospinal fluid from the fourth ventricle enters the subarachnoid space of the pontine cistern via these openings. The location of the foramina can be verified by gently inserting a blunt probe into the opening through which the choroid plexus is visible and directing the probe medially. Lift the medulla in order to view the cavity of the fourth ventricle through the foramen of Magendie and you will see the tip of the probe enter the ventricle.

3. The *interpeduncular cistern* overlies the ventral surface of the midbrain enclosing the cerebral peduncles and interpeduncular fossa (Fig. 8-4). This cistern is formed by the arachnoid bridging the gap between the temporal lobes of cerebral hemispheres. Anteriorly, it continues as a series of less prominent cisternae that include the *cistern of the optic chiasma,* the *cistern of the lamina terminalis,* and dorsally, the *cistern of the corpus callosum (supracallosal cistern)* lying between the free border of the falx cerebri and the dorsal surface of the corpus callosum.

4. The *cistern of the lateral sulcus* is formed by the arachnoid bridging over the legnth of the lateral sulcus (of Sylvius) on the lateral convex surface of the hemisphere.

5. The *superior cistern (cistern of the great cerebral vein)* is located between the splenium of the corpus callosum and the dorsal surface of the midbrain in the region of the free anterior margin of the tentorium cerebelli. It contains the great cerebral vein (of Galen) referred to earlier. The term *cisterna ambiens* is sometimes applied to the group of subarachnoid cisternae that completely encircle the midbrain.

6. The *lumbar cistern* located at the caudal end of the spinal cord is described with the spinal cord in Chapter 12.

Pia Mater

The *pia mater* is a thin vascular membrane that adheres closely to the surface of the brain and spinal cord. Unlike either the arachnoid or the dura, it follows the contour of the gyri and sulci. The pial investment of the brain cannot be easily identified. With the arachnoid removed, however, the pia may be seen as a smooth glistening membrane that reflects light when the specimen is properly positioned. Extensions of the pia mater surround blood vessels for variable distances as they enter the substance of the brain. Invaginations of vascular pia into the lateral, third, and fourth ventricles are covered by specialized epithelium to form the choroid plexuses.

Figure 4-4.   Sagittal view of hemisected head with brain *in situ* showing the location of the major subarachnoid cisterns.

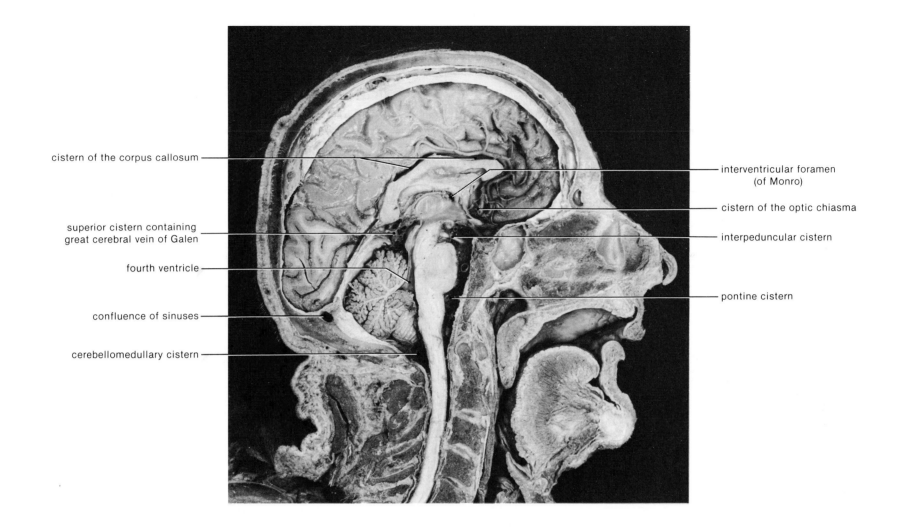

cistern of the corpus callosum

superior cistern containing
great cerebral vein of Galen

fourth ventricle

confluence of sinuses

cerebellomedullary cistern

interventricular foramen
(of Monro)

cistern of the optic chiasma

interpeduncular cistern

pontine cistern

5

Blood Supply of the Brain

The external cerebral arteries and veins lie in the subarachnoid space and are therefore partially concealed by the arachnoid where this is still present on the specimen. Wherever necessary, carefully strip the arachnoid away with forceps in order to follow the course of the vessels described below. In doing so, care must be taken to prevent tearing of the superficial cerebral veins, which are easily identified by their dark color, the coagulated and fixed venous blood being visible through their thin walls. Arteries have a paler appearance and are not easily torn because of their thicker muscular walls. Do not remove the arachnoid from around the brain stem. This will be accomplished in Chapter 10.

Arteries

The brain receives its blood supply from two pairs of large arteries, the *vertebral* and the *carotid arteries*. Although the two arterial systems are interconnected by anastomoses, functionally they are essentially separate. In general, the *vertebral system* of arteries supplies the spinal cord, posterior cerebrum, midbrain, pons, medulla, and cerebellum, whereas the carotid arteries supply the anterior and middle portions of the cerebrum and the diencephalon. Approximately 80% of the blood supply of the brain comes from the carotid arteries, whereas the remaining 20% derives from the vertebral arteries.

Vertebral–Basilar Distribution

The specimen should have attached to the ventral surface of the medulla a short length of the right and left vertebral arteries. The vertebral arteries arise from the right and left subclavian arteries. They reach the brain by ascending in the foramina transversaria of the upper six cervical vertebrae and enter the posterior cranial fossa through the foramen magnum. At the pontemedullary junction, the two vertebral arteries join to form the *basilar artery* (Fig. 5-1), which extends forward along a shallow midline groove (the basilar sulcus) on the ventral surface of the pons (Fig. 3-1). Along their intracranial course, the vertebral arteries give rise to the following major branches, which should now be identified and traced as far as possible.

1. The *anterior spinal artery* is located in the ventral or anterior median fissure of the medulla and spinal cord (Fig. 5-1). It is formed by the union of two branches, one from each vertebral artery, just before they merge to form the basilar artery. The vascular configuration thus formed has the shape of the letter Y. This single anterior spinal artery is reinforced by a series of radicular arteries along the length of the spinal cord. Small branches of the anterior spinal artery penetrate the spinal cord and supply the white matter of the ventral and lateral funiculi and the gray matter of the ventral horns, reaching as far as the base of the dorsal horns. The anterior spinal artery also supplies the ventromedial part of the medulla.

2. The *posterior spinal arteries* arise from either the vertebral or the posterior inferior cerebellar arteries. They each descend along the

---

Figure 5-1. Arteries of the base of the brain. The inset shows at higher magnification the arteries that compose the circle of Willis.

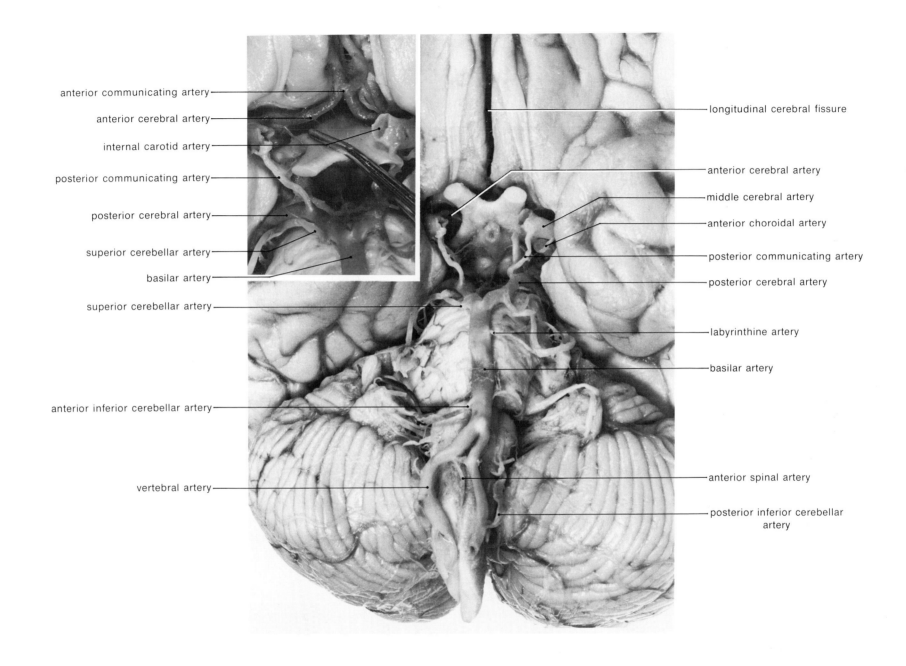

anterior communicating artery

anterior cerebral artery

internal carotid artery

posterior communicating artery

posterior cerebral artery

superior cerebellar artery

basilar artery

superior cerebellar artery

anterior inferior cerebellar artery

vertebral artery

longitudinal cerebral fissure

anterior cerebral artery

middle cerebral artery

anterior choroidal artery

posterior communicating artery

posterior cerebral artery

labyrinthine artery

basilar artery

anterior spinal artery

posterior inferior cerebellar artery

27

dorsolateral surface of the spinal cord, forming a plexiform channel along the line of attachment of the dorsal roots of the spinal nerves. As with the anterior spinal artery, the posterior spinal arteries are joined by a series of radicular arteries along the length of the cord. These arteries supply the white matter of the dorsal funiculi of the spinal cord and the dorsal horns.

3. The *posterior inferior cerebellar* arteries are the largest branches arising from the vertebral arteries. In favorable specimens having a long length of attached medulla, the posterior inferior cerebellar arteries may be seen to arise from the vertebral arteries at the level of the caudal end of the medulla (Fig. 5-1). They then pass dorsally and laterally around the medulla into the vallecula of the cerebellum to supply the inferior cerebellar peduncle and the posterior and inferior parts of the cerebellum. Small twigs are given off the trunk of the artery to the lateral medulla and the choroid plexus of the fourth ventricle. It is important to note that the region of the dorsolateral medulla (i.e., the area dorsal to the inferior olivary nucleus), which is supplied by the posterior inferior cerebellar artery, includes the spinothalamic tracts and the spinal nucleus and tract of the trigeminal nerve, among other structures. Occlusion of this artery, therefore, results in the *lateral medullary syndrome (Wallenberg's syndrome)*, which is characterized by loss of pain and thermal sensation on the ipsilateral side of the face and on the contralateral side of the body.

The following important arteries of the vertebral–basilar distribution, which should now be identified, all are branches arising from the basilar artery.

4. The *anterior inferior cerebellar artery* arises just after the vertebral arteries unite to form the basilar artery (Fig. 5-1). Follow it along the pontomedullary border and note that it is distributed to the anterior and inferior surfaces of the cerebellum. Along its course, a few small branches are given off to the lateral surface of the pons, the superior and middle cerebellar peduncles, the deep cerebellar nuclei, and the choroid plexus of the fourth ventricle.

5. The *labyrinthine* or *internal auditory artery* may arise directly from the basilar artery or, more frequently, as a branch from the anterior inferior cerebellar artery. In either case, it enters the internal acoustic meatus and supplies the cochlea and the vestibular portion of the inner ear.

6. A series of small paramedian and lateral *pontine arteries* emerge from the basilar artery as it runs along the length of the pons. They extend laterally for variable distances before penetrating the basilar portion of the pons. The *paramedian* branches, as their name implies, supply the most medial areas of the basilar pons and the ventral part of the pontine tegmentum. The structures supplied include the pontine nuclei, the corticospinal and corticobulbar tracts, and the medial lemniscus. The *lateral pontine* arteries can be classified into *short* and *long circumferential* branches. The short circumferential arteries extend farther laterally than do the paramedian arteries and supply the anterolateral region of the pons. The long circumferential branches extend still farther laterally, over the anterior surface of the pons, to supply the pontine tegmentum. Sudden occlusion of the basilar artery, although rare, may produce massive damage of important neural structures within the pons, which is usually fatal.

7. The *superior cerebellar artery* is the penultimate branch of the basilar artery, arising just below the emergence of the root of the oculomotor nerve from the interpeduncular fossa. It passes dorsolaterally around the cerebral peduncles and, as its name suggests, is distributed to the superior surface of the cerebellum. In addition, small branches are given off to the midbrain, the pons, the deep cerebellar nuclei, the superior cerebellar peduncle, the pineal gland, and the choroid plexus.

8. The *posterior cerebral arteries* are the terminal branches of the basilar artery, Just distal to the terminal bifurcation of the basilar, each posterior cerebral artery receives an anastomotic branch known as the posterior communicating artery from the internal carotid artery. Each posterior cerebral artery then curves around the midbrain, above the oculomotor and trochlear nerves, through the tentorial incisure and courses along the medial and inferior surface of the occipital and temporal lobes. By gentle dissection with the blunt probe, follow the course of this artery as far as possible. Its cortical branches supply the medial and inferior surface of the occipital lobe, the posterior part of the lateral surface of the occipital lobe, the inferior sur-

Figure 5-2. Lateral and ventromedial views of the cerebrum showing the cortical distribution of the anterior, middle, and posterior cerebral arteries. In this preparation, the meninges were removed and the arteries painted. The white line in the region of the parietooccipital sulcus illustrates the line of demarcation between anterior and posterior cerebral artery distributions.

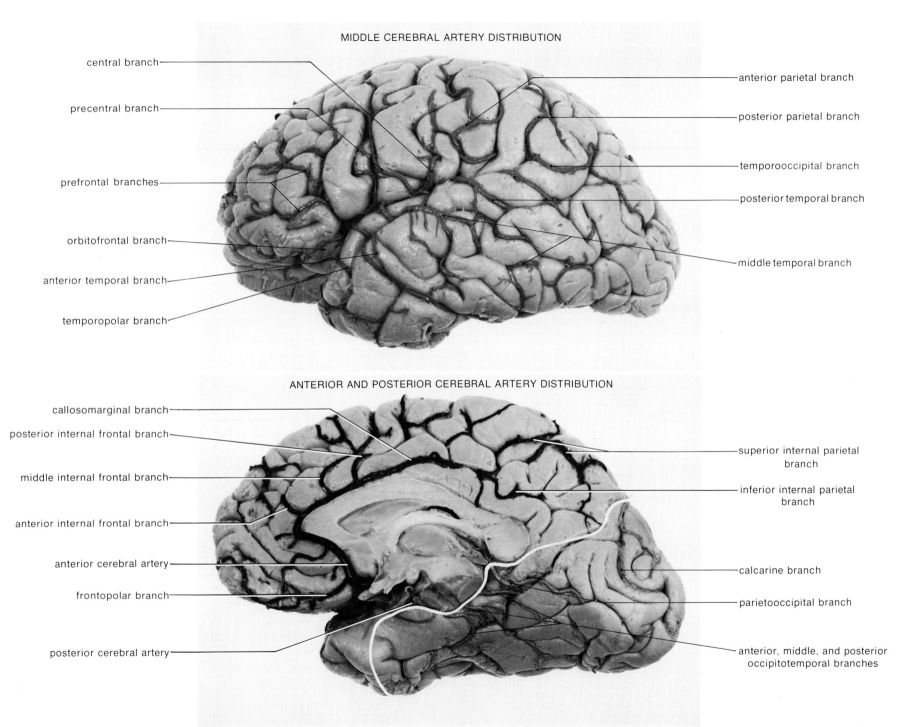

MIDDLE CEREBRAL ARTERY DISTRIBUTION

central branch

precentral branch

prefrontal branches

orbitofrontal branch

anterior temporal branch

temporopolar branch

anterior parietal branch

posterior parietal branch

temporooccipital branch

posterior temporal branch

middle temporal branch

ANTERIOR AND POSTERIOR CEREBRAL ARTERY DISTRIBUTION

callosomarginal branch

posterior internal frontal branch

middle internal frontal branch

anterior internal frontal branch

anterior cerebral artery

frontopolar branch

posterior cerebral artery

superior internal parietal branch

inferior internal parietal branch

calcarine branch

parietooccipital branch

anterior, middle, and posterior occipitotemporal branches

29

face of the temporal lobe (but not the temporal pole), and the lateral surface of the inferior temporal gyrus (Fig. 5-2). The primary visual area of the cerebral cortex is included in the area supplied by the posterior cerebral arteries. Branches of the posterior cerebral artery are also distributed to the choroid plexus of the lateral and third ventricles, the diencephalon, and the midbrain but cannot be identified at this stage of the dissection.

Carotid Distribution

The cut end of the large artery at the lateral edge of the optic chiasma is that of the *internal carotid artery* (Fig. 5-1). As stated in Chapter 4, this artery traverses the cavernous sinus for a short distance in its intracranial course. In so doing it gives off small branches that supply the trigeminal ganglion and the walls of the neighboring venous sinuses, as well as the important hypophysial vessels. These arteries will probably not be present in the specimen. However, the following major branches of the internal carotid artery, arising after it leaves the cavernous sinus, should now be identified.

1. The *ophthalmic artery* is the first major branch arising from the carotid after it leaves the cavernous sinus. The ophthalmic artery enters the orbit through the optic foramen of the skull and supplies the retina, the lacrimal glands, and many other structures contained within the orbital cavity.

2. The *posterior communicating artery* runs backward to anastomose with the posterior cerebral artery, which is the terminal branch of the basilar artery.

3. The *anterior choroidal artery* usually arises from the carotid artery just distal to the emergence of the posterior communicating artery (Fig. 5-1). Follow its course for a short distance as it passes backward along the optic tract to the medial surface of the temporal lobe. It enters the inferior horn of the lateral ventricle via the choroidal fissure and supplies the choroid plexus of the ventricle. Although the anterior choroidal artery is a relatively small vessel, it does supply a larger area of the brain than its name would imply. Branches are provided to the posterior limb and retrolenticular portions of the internal capsule, the globus pallidus, the lateral geniculate nucleus of the thalamus, and the hippocampal formation and amygdala in the temporal lobe. Occlusion of this long slender artery has widespread neurologic consequences.

4. The *anterior cerebral artery* (Fig. 5-1) arises from the carotid ar-

tery at the anteromedial end of the lateral sulcus. It proceeds forward and medially above the optic nerve to the longitudinal cerebral fissure. Along with its counterpart from the opposite side it disappears into the depths of this fissure by curving dorsally around the genu of the corpus callosum. By gently separating the frontal lobes one may be able to follow the anterior cerebral artery a short distance into the longitudinal fissure. Just anterior to the optic chiasma, the right and left anterior cerebral arteries approach each other. At this point they are joined together by a short artery called the *anterior communicating artery*. The cortical branches of the anterior cerebral arteries supply the medial surface of the cerebral hemisphere, including the corpus callosum, as far back as the parietooccipital sulcus. Branches of the anterior cerebral arteries extend over the superior convex border of the hemisphere to supply a narrow strip on the dorsolateral surface of the hemisphere that extends as far back as the parietooccipital sulcus (Fig. 5-2).

5. The *middle cerebral artery* is the largest branch of the internal carotid artery and is a continuation of the parent vessel. It passes laterally to enter the lateral sulcus, and you may view it by separating the opercular cortex on each side of the sulcus and looking down into its depths. Many branches that arise in the region of the insula emerge from the lateral sulcus to supply the lateral convex surface of the cerebral hemisphere, which includes large parts of the frontal and parietal lobe, the lateral surface of the temporal lobe including the temporal pole, and most of the lateral surface of the occipital lobe (Fig. 5-2). Note that although the middle cerebral artery provides the principal blood supply to the lateral surface of the hemispheres, it does not supply the whole of the lateral surface. Recall that both the anterior and posterior cerebral arteries are reflected onto the lateral surface of the hemispheres in certain locations, as already indicated. Because of the many important areas of cortex supplied by the middle cerebral artery—areas that will be examined in the following chapter—its occlusion results in grave sensory and motor deficits, which may include the faculty of language if the dominant hemisphere is affected.

Cerebral Arterial Circle (of Willis)

The arterial circle of Willis, located at the base of the brain, is formed by a series of anastomosing vessels that link the internal carotid and the vertebral–basilar distributions. It is formed in front by the *ante-*

rior communicating and paired anterior cerebral arteries, and behind by the *paired carotids, posterior communicating, and posterior cerebral arteries* (Fig. 5-1).

Central (Ganglionic) Arteries

Many fine arterial branches arise from the proximal parts of the anterior, middle, and posterior cerebral arteries and the arterial circle of Willis. They are referred to as *central* or *ganglionic* branches because they penetrate the surface of the brain to supply the corpus striatum, diencephalon, internal capsule, and parts of the midbrain. Four groups of central arteries are usually distinguished, although they are small and not easily identified. If they cannot be found on the specimen, consult a text for their precise location and distribution.

1. The *anteromedial group*. These small arteries are derived from the anterior communicating artery and from a short segment of the anterior cerebral artery immediately after it leaves the carotid artery. They curve medially and abruptly penetrate the thin layer of cortex just superior and rostral to the optic chiasma, in an area known as the anterior perforated substance (Fig. 8-4). These arteries supply the anterior portions of the hypothalamus, putamen, and caudate nuclei.

2. The *anterolateral group*. These arteries originate mainly from the proximal end of the middle cerebral artery and penetrate the anterior perforated substance at its lateral border. They are also referred to as the *striate arteries* because they supply most of the corpus striatum. In addition, they also supply the lateral hypothalamus and most of the internal capsule.

3. The *posteromedial group*. These arteries are medially directed branches arising from the posterior communicating and posterior cerebral arteries. They pierce the surface of the brain stem in the interpeduncular fossa just behind the mamillary bodies in the same manner as those of the anteromedial group. This area is therefore called the *posterior perforated substance*. These arteries supply regions of the hypothalamus, subthalamus, anteromedial thalamus, and the cerebral peduncles.

4. The *posterolateral group*. These central arteries arises from the posterior cerebral artery lateral to the posterior communicating artery. They are distributed to the posterior thalamus, pineal gland, midbrain tectum, and cerebral peduncles.

Veins

The cerebral veins are usually divided into *external* and *internal groups*. The *external cerebral veins* drain blood from the surface, that is, the cortex and outer regions of the subcortical white matter of the hemispheres. They empty into the superior sagittal sinus or the transverse and cavernous sinuses. The *internal group of cerebral veins* drains deeper structures within the interior of the cerebral hemispheres such as the basal ganglia, the diencephalon, and the choroid plexuses. They eventually empty into the great cerebral vein (of Galen) and the straight sinus. The internal cerebral veins are periventricular in location and will be seen in the course of the dissection of the interior of the hemisphere (Chapter 8). Both groups of cerebral veins differ from other veins of the body in that they have thinner walls and do not possess valves. An attempt should now be made to identify the following external cerebral veins located within the subarachnoid space:

1. The *superior cerebral veins* are 8 to 15 in number. They pursue a tortuous course along the sulci toward the superior border of the hemisphere. They drain the lateral convexity and medial surface of the hemisphere and open obliquely into the superior sagittal sinus (Fig. 5-3).

2. The *superficial middle cerebral vein* extends obliquely over the lateral surface of the hemisphere downward and forward within the subarachnoid space of the lateral sulcus. At the temporal pole it turns medially to open directly into the cavernous sinus. The superficial middle cerebral vein is linked to the superior sagittal sinus by the *superior anastomotic vein (of Trolard)*, which runs over the lateral surface of the cortex. In a similar fashion, the *superficial middle cerebral vein* is joined with the transverse sinus by the *inferior anastomotic vein (of Labbé)*, which courses backward over the temporal lobe. The superior sagittal, transverse, and cavernous sinuses are thus linked by these two anastomotic veins.

3. The *deep middle cerebral vein* receives blood from the insula and neighboring regions of the cortex and follows a ventrally directed course similar to that of the superificial middle cerebral vein, described previously. It lies deep within the floor of the lateral sulcus, however, and may be seen only if you gently separate the lips of the lateral sulcus and look into its depths. Its darker color distinguishes the vein from the middle cerebral artery.

4. Numerous small inferior cerebral veins drain the ventral and

lower lateral surfaces of the hemispheres. They ultimately empty into the cavernous sinus by means of the superior petrosal and transverse sinuses. These will probably not be present on the brain specimen.

5. The *basal vein (of Rosenthal)* begins at the base of the hemisphere near the anterior perforated substance, where it is formed by the union of the anterior cerebral and deep middle cerebral veins. It courses backward toward the interpeduncular fossa of the midbrain and curves around the cerebral peduncle to join the great cerebral vein (of Galen). Although the basal vein may not be present in the brain specimen, you will be able to identify the latter vein in a subsequent dissection.

6. The *anterior cerebral vein* is located on the medial surface of the hemisphere. It follows a course similar to that of its arterial counterpart, and you may see it by separating the two frontal lobes and looking into the depths of the longitudinal cerebral fissure.

In addition to the cerebral veins described in the foregoing section, there are also cerebellar veins and veins of the brain stem that drain into dural venous sinuses at the base of the skull.

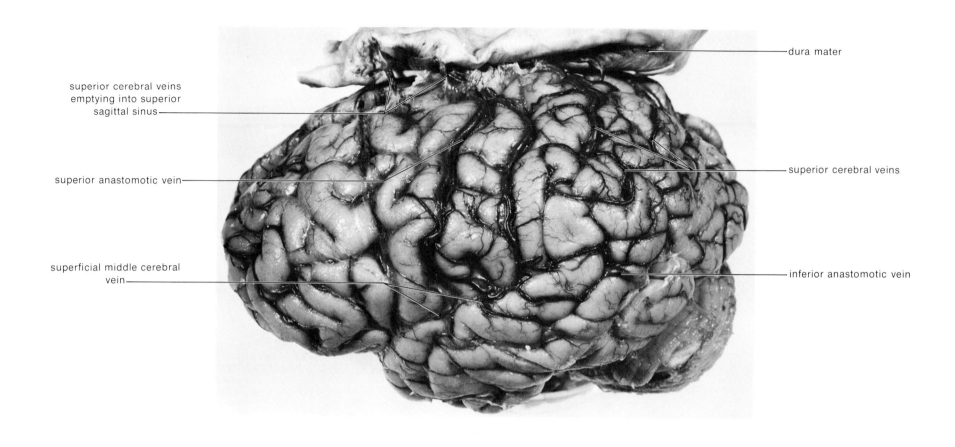

superior cerebral veins emptying into superior sagittal sinus

dura mater

superior cerebral veins

superior anastomotic vein

superficial middle cerebral vein

inferior anastomotic vein

Figure 5-3. Lateral view of the brain showing the superficial cerebral veins.

6

Topography of the Cerebral Hemispheres

The meninges and the superficial vessels of the cerebrum should now be removed. This is accomplished by stripping them away from the surface with fingers and forceps. The end result is a clear and unobstructed view of the arrangement of gyri and sulci on the surface of the hemisphere (see Fig. 6-2). Do not remove the meninges from the brain stem at this time.

Examine the right and left *cerebral hemispheres*. In lower mammals such as rodents, the surface of the cerebral hemisphere is devoid of convolutions. Such brains are referred to as *lissencephalic*. In higher mammals, especially primates, the surface of the hemispheres assumes a highly convoluted pattern to permit a great surface area and volume of cortical gray matter without the necessity of a corresponding increase in the size of the cranial cavity. Such brains are called *gyrencephalic*. The convolutions on the surface of the human cerebrum are called *gyri* (singular: *gyrus*) and the grooves or troughs between them are called *sulci* (singular: *sulcus*). At one time large and deep sulci were called *fissures*. However, modern neuroanatomic terminology restricts the use of this word to the description of large clefts that form in its development between one part of the brain and another. Examples are the *longitudinal cerebral fissure* and the *transverse cerebral fissure*. Locate the following fissures and sulci on the specimen with the assistance of Figures 6-1 through 6-6.

1. The *longitudinal cerebral fissure* is a deep fissure running anteoposteriorly in the midline that incompletely divides the cerebrum into left and right hemispheres (Fig. 6-1). At the base of the longitudinal fissure is the corpus callosum, a stout band of white matter that interconnects the hemispheres. The corpus callosum will be examined in detail in Chapter 7.

2. The *lateral sulcus* (of Sylvius) is a deep groove that begins at the inferior surface of the hemisphere above the temporal pole and courses obliquely backward and upward along the lateral convex surface of the hemisphere (Figs. 6-2 and 6-4). Near its beginning, two short rami of the lateral sulcus project into the frontal lobe; these are the *ascending* and the *anterior rami*. The ascending ramus projects upward into the frontal lobe (Fig. 6-2). The anterior ramus arises from the same point as the ascending ramus but projects almost horizontally toward the frontal pole (the most rostral tip of the hemisphere). Unfortunately, the brain specimen shown in Figure 6-2 does not have a prominent anterior ramus. The remainder of the lateral sulcus continues posteriorly as the *posterior ramus* (Fig. 6-2).

3. The *central sulcus* (of Rolando) begins at the superior border of the hemisphere slightly behind the midpoint between the frontal and occipital poles (Figs. 6-1 and 6-4). It descends with a slight forward inclination across the lateral surface of the hemisphere to approach (but not quite reach) the posterior ramus of the lateral sulcus at an acute angle (Fig. 6-2). Insert the blunt end of the scalpel handle into the sulcus to obtain some appreciation of its depth.

4. The *parietooccipital sulcus* is found on the medial surface of the hemisphere (Figs. 6-3 and 6-5). You may see it by spreading the posterior ends of the cerebral hemispheres and looking at the medial surface of one side. It begins at the superior border about 4–5

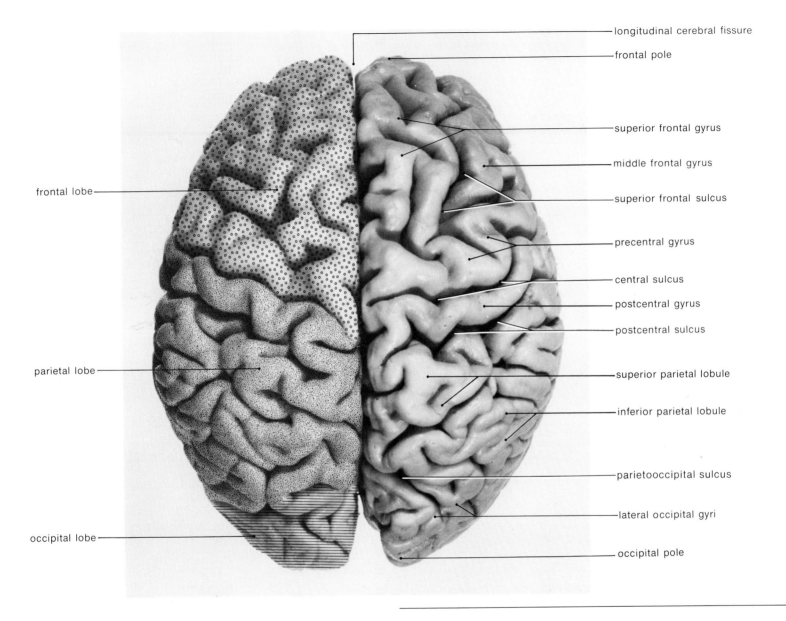

longitudinal cerebral fissure

frontal pole

superior frontal gyrus

middle frontal gyrus

superior frontal sulcus

precentral gyrus

central sulcus

postcentral gyrus

postcentral sulcus

superior parietal lobule

inferior parietal lobule

parietooccipital sulcus

lateral occipital gyri

occipital pole

frontal lobe

parietal lobe

occipital lobe

Figure 6-1. View of the superior surface of the brain. The extent of the frontal, parietal, and occipital lobes is demonstrated in the left hemisphere. The gyri and sulci are indicated in the right hemisphere.

35

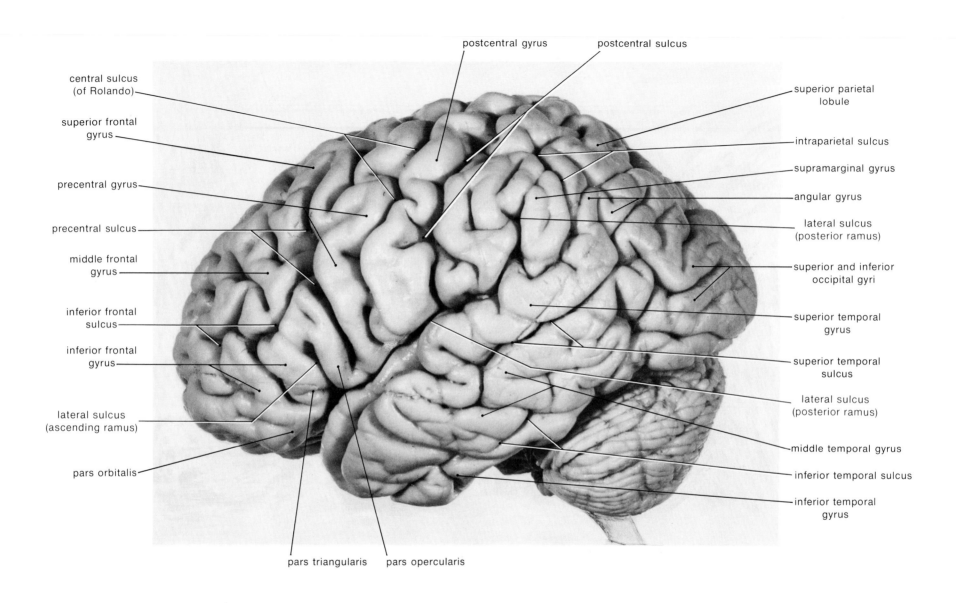

central sulcus
(of Rolando)

superior frontal
gyrus

precentral gyrus

precentral sulcus

middle frontal
gyrus

inferior frontal
sulcus

inferior frontal
gyrus

lateral sulcus
(ascending ramus)

pars orbitalis

pars triangularis   pars opercularis

postcentral gyrus   postcentral sulcus

superior parietal
lobule

intraparietal sulcus

supramarginal gyrus

angular gyrus

lateral sulcus
(posterior ramus)

superior and inferior
occipital gyri

superior temporal
gyrus

superior temporal
sulcus

lateral sulcus
(posterior ramus)

middle temporal gyrus

inferior temporal sulcus

inferior temporal
gyrus

Figure 6-2. Gyri and sulci on the lateral surface of the cerebral hemisphere.

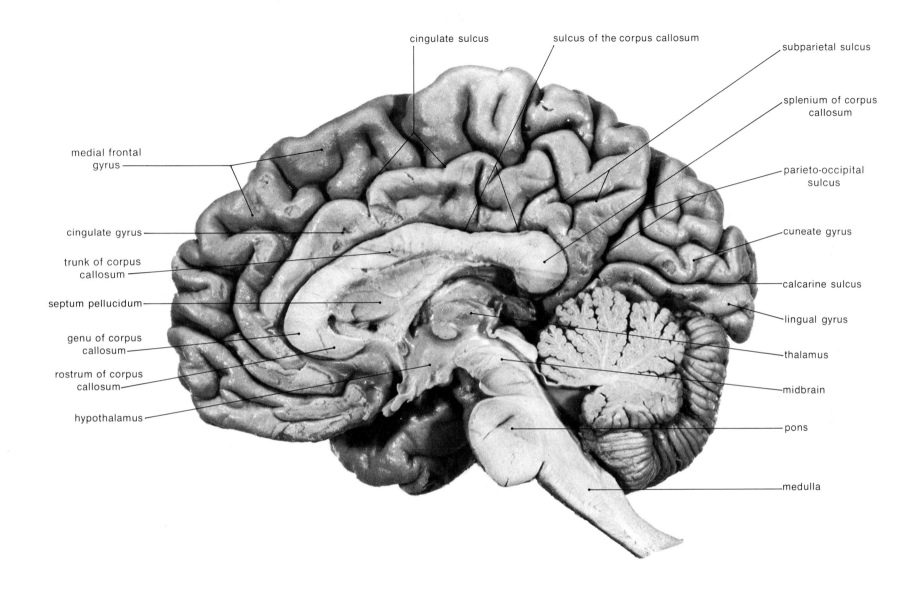

cingulate sulcus

sulcus of the corpus callosum

subparietal sulcus

splenium of corpus callosum

medial frontal gyrus

parieto-occipital sulcus

cingulate gyrus

cuneate gyrus

trunk of corpus callosum

calcarine sulcus

septum pellucidum

lingual gyrus

genu of corpus callosum

thalamus

rostrum of corpus callosum

midbrain

hypothalamus

pons

medulla

Figure 6-3. Medial view of the right half of a brain sectioned in the sagittal plane to demonstrate the gyri and sulci on the medial surface of the hemisphere.

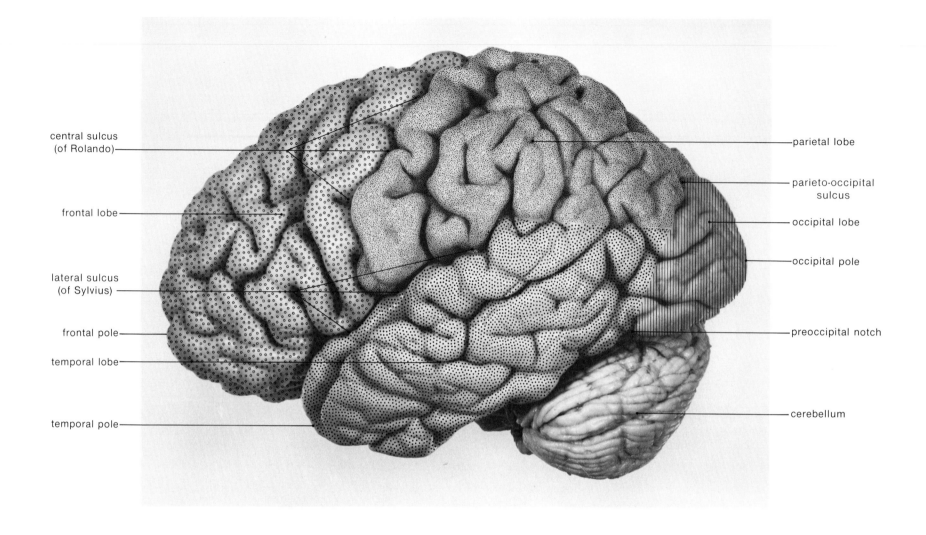

central sulcus
(of Rolando)

frontal lobe

lateral sulcus
(of Sylvius)

frontal pole

temporal lobe

temporal pole

parietal lobe

parieto-occipital
sulcus

occipital lobe

occipital pole

preoccipital notch

cerebellum

Figure 6-4. Lateral view of the brain demonstrating the various lobes of the hemisphere.

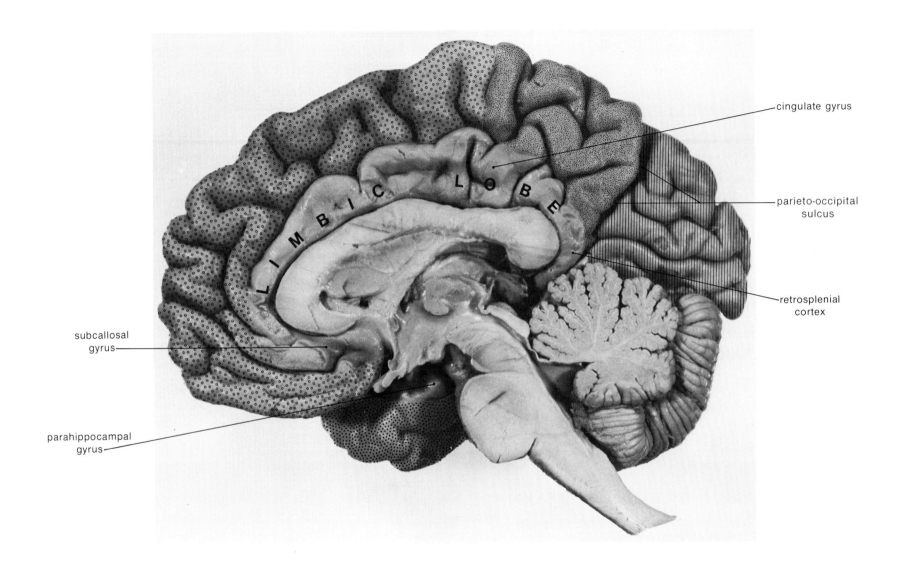

cingulate gyrus

parieto-occipital
sulcus

retrosplenial
cortex

subcallosal
gyrus

parahippocampal
gyrus

Figure 6-5. Right half of a hemisected brain showing the lobes of the brain as seen on the medial surface of the hemisphere.

39

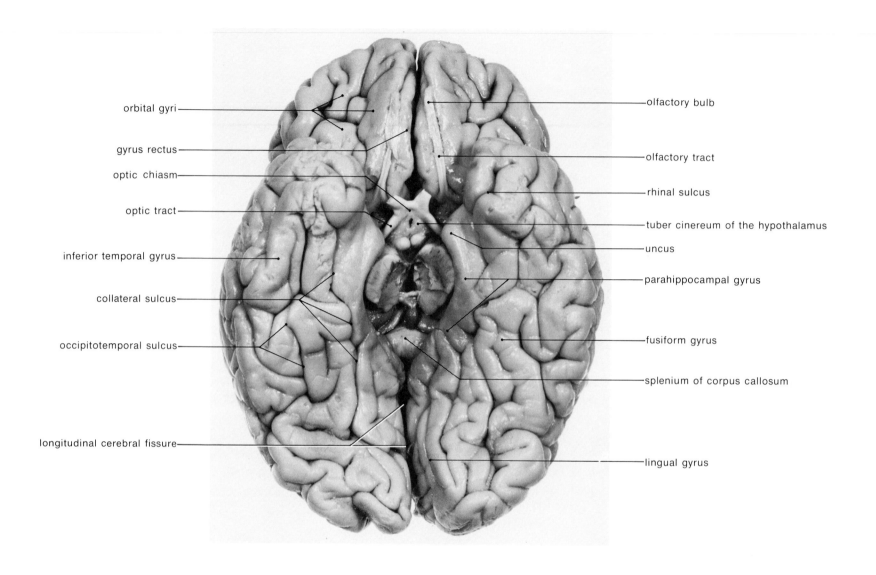

orbital gyri

gyrus rectus

optic chiasm

optic tract

inferior temporal gyrus

collateral sulcus

occipitotemporal sulcus

longitudinal cerebral fissure

olfactory bulb

olfactory tract

rhinal sulcus

tuber cinereum of the hypothalamus

uncus

parahippocampal gyrus

fusiform gyrus

splenium of corpus callosum

lingual gyrus

Figure 6-6. Inferior surface of the brain after transection of the midbrain to remove the brain stem and cerebellum.

cm in front of the occipital pole (the most caudal tip of the hemisphere) and courses obliquely downward and forward to join the calcarine sulcus. This sulcus is reflected for a short distance over the superior border of the hemisphere onto the lateral surface (Figs. 6-1 and 6-4).

The landmarks just described form the boundaries of regions called lobes, into which the hemispheres are divided. They are the *frontal lobe, parietal lobe, occipital lobe,* and *temporal lobe* (Figs. 6-1 and 6-4). In addition, a large area on the medial surface of the hemisphere that is composed of parts of the above lobes is usually regarded as constituting a separate lobe, the *limbic lobe* (Fig. 6-5). A description of the limbic lobe is found in Chapter 9.

The lobes of the brain themselves are divided into lobules and gyri by shallow *sulci.* There is a good deal of variation in the configuration of these gyri and sulci from one brain to another and even between the two hemispheres of the one brain. Examine the brain specimens of the students groups near you in order to gain some appreciation of the degree of variation.

Now examine the lobes of the hemisphere in more detail.

1. The *frontal lobe* is that part of the hemisphere rostral to the central sulcus and superior to the lateral sulcus (Figs. 6-1 and 6-4). It is the largest lobe of the hemisphere. Its most rostral limit is the *frontal pole.* On its lateral surface, running parallel with the central sulcus but also 1.5 cm in front of it, is the *precentral sulcus* (Fig. 6-2). The *precentral gyrus* is the convolution that lies between these two sulci. In front of the precentral sulcus and running at a right angle to it are two horizontally directed sulci. They are the *superior frontal sulcus* (Fig. 6-1), close to the superiomedial border of the lobe, and the *inferior frontal sulcus* (Fig. 6-2), located approximately midway between the superior and inferior borders. These sulci form the boundaries of three gyri: the *superior, middle,* and *inferior frontal gyri.* The ascending and anterior rami of the lateral sulcus divide the inferior frontal gyrus into three portions called the *pars orbitalis,* the *pars triangularis,* and the *pars opercularis* (Fig. 6-2). The structures on the inferior or orbital surface of the frontal lobe will be described later.

2. The *parietal lobe* is bounded in front by the central sulcus, below by the posterior ramus of the lateral sulcus, and behind by an imaginary line extending from the parietooccipital sulcus on the superior border of the hemisphere to the *preoccipital notch* on the inferior surface (Figs. 6-1 and 6-4). The preoccipital notch is a small indentation produced by the petrous temporal bone on the inferolateral border of the hemisphere about 4 cm in front of the occipital pole. Once again paralleling the central sulcus, but this time about 1 cm behind it, is the *postcentral sulcus* (Figs. 6-1 and 6-2). This may not be a continuous sulcus, for it is frequently interrupted by intervening gyri. Between this sulcus and the central sulcus is the *postcentral gyrus.* Immediately behind the postcentral gyrus and roughly at right angle to it is the *intraparietal sulcus,* which curves for a distance of 4–6 cm toward the occipital pole. This sulcus is irregular and frequently broken by gyri bridging across it. It divides the parietal lobe into the *superior parietal lobule* above and the *inferior parietal lobule* below (Figs. 6-1 and 6-2). The inferior parietal lobule consists of two gyri. The *supramarginal gyrus* surrounds the upturned end of the posterior ramus of the lateral sulcus, and the *angular gyrus* surrounds the upturned posterior end of the superior temporal sulcus.

3. The small *occipital lobe* is a triangular portion of the hemisphere located behind the imaginary line joining the parietooccipital sulcus with the preoccipital notch (Fig. 6-4). Its posterior limit is the *occipital pole.* On the lateral surface of the occipital lobe there is usually a short horizontal sulcus, the *lateral occipital sulcus,* which divides the lateral surface of the lobe into *superior* and inferior *occipital gyri* (Fig. 6-2). These minor markings on the lateral convex surface of the lobe are irregular and not always present. Spread the hemispheres apart to examine the medial surface of the occipital lobe. More of the occipital lobe is visible on the medial surface of the hemisphere. The *calcarine sulcus* is a horizontal groove that extends from the occipital pole forward to a point just below the splenium of the corpus callosum. It is joined by the vertical parietooccipital sulcus at an acute angle to form a Y-shaped configuration. The gyrus below the calcarine sulcus is the *lingual gyrus,* and the one above is the *cuneate gyrus* (Fig. 6-3).

4. The *temporal lobe* is located along the inferior aspect of the hemisphere below the frontal and parietal lobes and is separated from them by the lateral sulcus. Its posterior boundary is the imaginary line referred to earlier, joining the parietooccipital sulcus with the preoccipital notch (Fig. 6-4). The most rostral limit of this lobe is the *temporal pole.* Below the posterior ramus of the lateral sulcus and running parallel to it are two sulci, the *superior* and *inferior temporal sulci.* The superior temporal sulcus is usually a continuous sul-

cus located 1.0–1.5 cm below the lateral sulcus. Its posterior end curves upward into the parietal lobe (Fig. 6-2). The inferior temporal sulcus lies at the inferolateral border of the lobe. It is usually broken up into two or three short sulci by intervening gyri, but posteriorly it also ascends into the parietal lobe. These sulci divide the lateral surface of the temporal lobe into three gyri: the *superior, middle,* and *inferior temporal gyri.* Spread the lips of the lateral sulcus with fingers and thumb and examine the broad dorsomedial surface of the superior temporal gyrus. Note at least two gyri running obliquely across this surface; they are the *transverse temporal gyri.* The inferior surface of the temporal lobe can be seen better if the brain stem and cerebellum are removed. This is accomplished as follows: Turn the brain so that the right and left occipital poles face you. Separate the cerebrum from the cerebellum by exerting a gentle pressure on them. Look down into the space between them and note the tangle of vascular meninges. This is the *pia-arachnoid* of the *transverse cerebral fissure,* which will be described later in Chapter 9. By blunt dissection with a probe, free the arachnoid from the surface of the midbrain. The *pineal gland* will be seen enclosed within the pia-arachnoid in the dorsal midline (see Fig. 13-1). On the dorsal surface of the midbrain identify two pairs of small elevations (the corpora quadrigemina); these are the *superior colliculi* and the *inferior colliculi.* Using the blade of a scalpel, make bilateral transverse incisions through the dorsal brain stem just rostral to the superior colliculi. Now turn the brain over so that the ventral surface faces you and locate the cerebral peduncles of the midbrain and the mamillary bodies of the hypothalamus (see Fig. 3-1 to locate these structures). Complete the transection of the midbrain by cutting through the peduncles just behind the mamillary bodies. Store the brain stem and cerebellum thus removed. This maneuver must be done correctly; if there is doubt about the landmarks, consult an instructor.

Having removed the brain stem and cerebellum from the cerebrum, you will now be able to view the structures on the ventral (inferior) surface of the hemisphere to better advantage (Fig. 6-6). Identify the *olfactory bulb* and the *olfactory tract,* which lie in the *olfactory sulcus* on each side of the longitudinal cerebral fissure at the base of the frontal lobes. The strip of cortex between the olfactory sulcus and the longitudinal fissure is the *gyrus rectus* or *straight gyrus.* The remainder of the orbital surface of the frontal lobe lateral to the olfactory sulcus consists of several small irregular gyri known collectively as the *orbital gyri.*

The gyri on the inferior surface of the temporal lobe are arranged in a longitudinal direction. The sulci between the gyri are often irregular and discontinuous. The most medial of the gyri is the *parahippocampal gyrus* (Fig. 6-6), which extends forward from the lingual gyrus at the level of the isthmus where it blends with the cingulate gyrus that curves behind and above the corpus callosum (see Figs. 6-3 and 6-5). The small hooklike convolution on its anteromedial border, which overlies the optic tract, is the *uncus.* The *collateral sulcus* marks the lateral border of the parahippocampal gyrus; it is usually interrupted along its length. The anterior extension of the collateral sulcus toward the temporal pole is the *rhinal sulcus.* Between the collateral sulcus and the more lateral *occipitotemporal sulcus* is the *fusiform* or *occipitotemporal gyrus* (Fig. 6-6).

Insula

Now orient the brain so that the lateral convex surface of the right hemisphere faces you, that is, the right frontal pole is to the right. Before exposing the insula, examine Figures 6-7 and 6-8. The insula is buried deep within the lateral sulcus hidden from view by parts of the frontal and parietal lobes. These parts are called the *frontal* and *parietal opercula* (operculum; from the Latin meaning a cover or lid). Grasp the scalpel so that the tip of the middle finger is not more than 3.5 cm from the tip of the scalpel blade. Insert the scalpel into the right hemisphere where the lateral sulcus begins to curve upward into the parietal lobe using the middle finger as a stop. With a short sawing motion make a semicircular cut ending at about the level of the temporal pole (Fig. 6-7). This cut should not be more than 3.5 cm deep and must not extend more than one-half the distance between the lateral sulcus and the superior border of the hemisphere. The parietal and frontal opercula will then easily come away from the rest of the hemisphere providing an unobstructed view of the transverse temporal gyri on the dorsal and medial surface of the temporal lobe (Fig. 6-8). It also exposes a region of cortex called the *insula* or *Island of Reil.* The insula is pyramidal in shape with its apex directed downward and forward in the lateral sulcus. The apex of the insula located near the stem of the lateral sulcus, where the insular cortex is continuous with that of the frontal lobe, is called the *limen insulae* (limen: from the Latin meaning the threshold or beginning). The cortex of the insula is usually divided into three anterior *short gyri* and two posterior *long gyri* by the *central sulcus of the insula.*

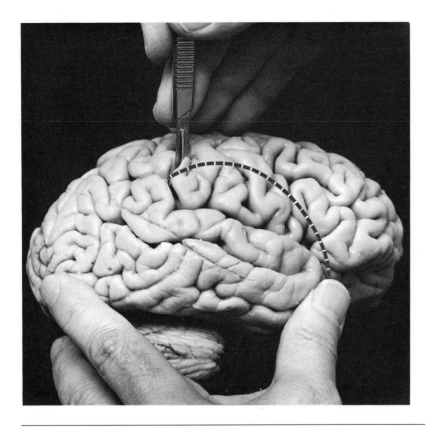

Figure 6-7.   Lateral view of the right hemisphere showing the technique for removing the frontal and parietal opercula.

Remove the superior portion of the right hemisphere by making successive horizontal slices with a long brain knife, each about 1 cm in thickness. The last cut should be 1.5 cm above the upper surface of the corpus callosum. This procedure exposes the medial surface of the left hemisphere (Fig. 6-9). Remove the arachnoid and any remaining blood vessels from the medial surface of the left hemisphere. Immediately above the corpus callosum, forming a line of demarcation between it and the cortex above, is a shallow sulcus known as the *sulcus of the corpus callosum* (Figs. 6-3 and 6-9). Between this sulcus and the superior border of the hemisphere is a parallel sulcus

that begins in front of and below the rostral end of the corpus callosum and curves upward and backward to indent the superior border of the hemisphere just behind the midpoint between the frontal and occipital poles. This is the *cingulate sulcus,* and the posterior upturned end is the *marginal ramus* (Figs. 6-9 and 13-1). The gyrus between the callosal and cingulate sulci just described is the *cingulate gyrus.* The cingulate gyrus and the parahippocampal gyrus are components of the *limbic lobe* (Chapter 9).

The cingulate sulcus also gives rise to the vertically directed *paracental sulcus,* which ascends to the superior border of the hemisphere at the level of the precentral sulcus about 4 cm in front of the marginal ramus (Fig. 6-9). The *subparietal sulcus* (Fig. 6-3) is the posterior continuation of the cingulate sulcus above the splenium of the corpus callosum to the parietooccipital sulcus. The two sulci are usually discontinuous, however. The area of cortex bounded by the parietooccipital sulcus, the subparietal sulcus, and the marginal ramus of the cingulate sulcus is called the *precuneus.* The cortical area located between the marginal ramus, the cingulate sulcus, and the paracentral sulcus is the *paracentral lobule.* Rostral to this is the *medial frontal gyrus* Figs. 6-3, 6-9 and 13-1). The gyri and sulci on the medial surface of the occipital lobe have been identified previously.

Cerebral Localization of Function

Special functions can be associated with certain areas of the cerebral cortex. Recall that there are differences in the histologic structure of the cortex from place to place and that there is, to a limited degree, some correlation between histologic structure and function. Review the histology of the cerebral cortex if necessary.

A number of regional maps of the cortex based on distinctive differences in structure have been produced. The cytoarchitectonic map of the cortex produced by Brodmann is still widely cited in clinical neurology, mainly for convenience. Figure 6-10 illustrates some of the important functional areas of the cerebral cortex and relates them to the Brodmann numbers referred to most frequently. With the assistance of this illustration, locate the following areas:

The *primary motor area* (area 4) is located in the precentral gyrus and includes the anterior paracentral lobule on the medial surface of the hemisphere.

The *premotor area* (area 6) is a strip of cortex located immediately in front of area 4 on both the lateral and medial surfaces of the

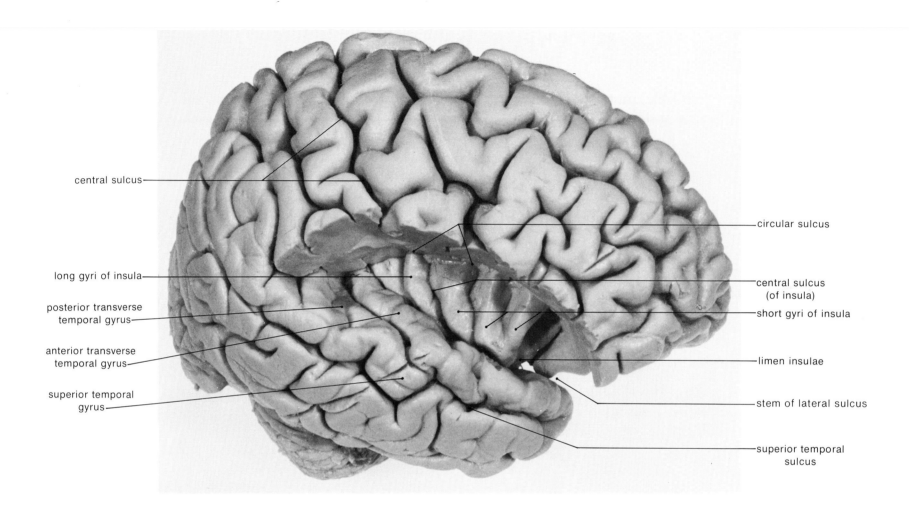

central sulcus

circular sulcus

long gyri of insula

central sulcus
(of insula)

posterior transverse
temporal gyrus

short gyri of insula

anterior transverse
temporal gyrus

limen insulae

superior temporal
gyrus

stem of lateral sulcus

superior temporal
sulcus

Figure 6-8. Lateral view of the right cerebral hemisphere showing the superior surface of the temporal lobe and the insula exposed by the removal of the frontal and parietal opercula.

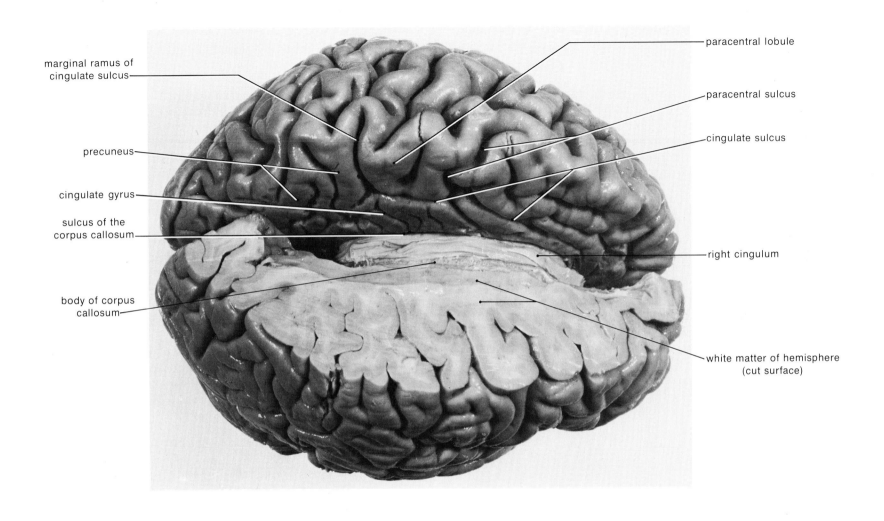

marginal ramus of
cingulate sulcus

precuneus

cingulate gyrus

sulcus of the
corpus callosum

body of corpus
callosum

paracentral lobule

paracentral sulcus

cingulate sulcus

right cingulum

white matter of hemisphere
(cut surface)

Figure 6-9. Dissection of the right cerebral hemisphere to demonstrate the right cingulum and the cortex of the medial surface of the left hemisphere.

frontal lobe. It includes the caudal part of the superior frontal gyrus and the rostral part of the precentral gyrus.

Cortical area 8 is located in the caudal portions of the superior and middle frontal gyri immediately rostral to area 6. The lower part of area 8, in the middle gyrus, is the *frontal eye field*, an area that controls voluntary conjugate movements of the eyes.

Broca's area (areas 44 and 45) is located in the caudal part of the inferior frontal gyrus (pars opercularis and triangularis). This area in the dominant hemisphere (usually the left) is responsible for the motor control of speech.

The *primary somesthetic area* (areas 3, 1, and 2) is located in the cortex of the postcentral gyrus and the caudal paracentral lobule. Area 3 occupies the posterior wall of the central sulcus and is more extensive than would appear from the dorsolateral surface. Area 2 is located along the posterior wall of the postcentral gyrus, and area 1 is interposed between the two. All three areas extend over the superiomedial border of the postcentral gyrus onto the paracentral lobule on the medial surface of the hemisphere. Impulses for the general sensations of pain, temperature, touch, pressure, and proprioception conveyed via the spinothalamic and trigeminothalamic tracts and the medial lemniscus ultimately reach this area.

The *gustatory area* (area 43) is believed to be located in the ventral part of the postcentral gyrus in the parietal operculum.

The *primary auditory area* (areas 41 and 42) is located in portions of the two anterior transverse temporal gyri (Heschl's convolutions) within the depths of the lateral sulcus.

The *visual (striate) area* (area 17) is located in the cortex (cuneate and lingual gyri) surrounding the calcarine sulcus of the occipital lobe.

The *sensory* or *ideational language area* (areas 40, 39, 22, and 21) is located within the complex of gyri formed by the supramarginal and angular gyri and the caudal portions of the superior and middle temporal gyri. The sensory language area is usually in the left hemisphere, which is the dominant hemisphere for language in most persons.

The *primary olfactory area* (area 34) is located in the temporal lobe cortex overlying the amygdaloid nucleus and the uncus.

Recently an area of the cerebral cortex has been identified as being related to the conscious appreciation of vestibular stimulation. It is located in the superior temporal gyrus just caudal to the auditory area in both hemispheres. It would include parts of Brodmann's areas 22, 39, and 40.

The terms associations areas of cortex and silent areas of cortex refer to those areas not having a primary sensory or motor function. The very use of these two terms (association and silent) betrays our lack of knowledge of precise functions of these large cortical areas. It is said that they provide for several characteristics peculiar to primates and to humans especially. They provide the means by which behavior can be controlled by an intellectual overlay based on judgment and reason.

Association areas of the frontal lobe (areas 9, 10, 11, 44, and 45) occupy most of the superior, middle, and inferior frontal gyri. Destructive lesions here result in behavioral changes in which the individual no longer seems concerned about the consequences of his actions or speech.

Association areas of the parietal lobe (areas 5, 7, 40, and 39) are contained within the superior and inferior parietal lobules and the precuneus on the medial surface of the hemisphere. Destructive lesions in the superior parietal lobule (areas 5 and 7) on one side may result in neglect of the opposite side of the body. Such individuals may very well deny that it belongs to them.

Visual association areas (areas 18 and 19) are located on each side of the calcarine sulcus adjacent to area 17 in the cuneate gyrus above and the lingual gyrus below. Areas 18 and 19 are related to smooth tracking movements of the eyes in conjunction with visual stimuli. These areas are sometimes referred to as the *occipital eye field.*

The auditory association area (area 22) is located behind the primary auditory area in the floor of the lateral sulcus (*planum temporale*) and includes parts of the superior temporal gyrus on the lateral surface of the temporal lobe. The auditory association cortex thus described is also known as *Wernicke's area.* Destructive lesions here result in receptive (sensory) aphasia, which is characterized by the individual's inability to understand the meaning of words in oral language.

Figure 6-10.   Lateral and medial views of the cerebral hemisphere illustrating the areas of localization of function using the map of Brodmann.

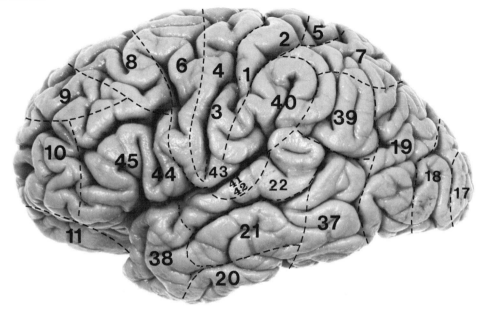

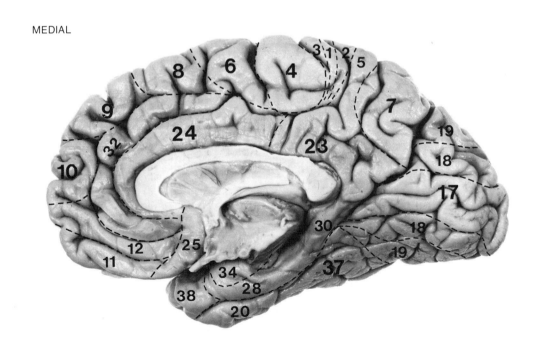

7

White Matter of the Cerebral Hemispheres and Basal Ganglia

The subcortical white matter of the cerebral hemisphere, sometimes referred to as the *medullary center*, is also called the *centrum semiovale* because of its semioval appearance when the hemisphere is sectioned horizontally. The central core of the hemisphere consists of a mass of intermingling fibers, most of which are myelinated and which are organized in bundles, or fasciculi, running in many directions. Fibers of the subcortical white matter can be classified according to the following three categories:

1. *Association fibers* are those that are wholly confined to one hemisphere. Short association fibers interconnect cortical areas of adjacent gyri, whereas long association fibers interconnect cortical areas that are further removed from each other, that is, in different lobes of the same hemisphere.

2. *Commissural fibers* originate from neuronal cell bodies in the cortex of one hemisphere; they cross the midline and synapse with neurons in areas of the cortex in the opposite hemisphere. In addition to the major commissures of the cerebral hemispheres, there are several small commissures that extend between corresponding nuclei in both halves of the brain stem.

3. *Projection* or *itinerant fibers* connect the cortex of the cerebrum with various subcortical loci and are of two types that are distinguished not on the basis of their gross morphology but on the basis of the direction of conduction. Afferent or *corticipetal fibers* arise mainly from neurons in the thalamus and project to the cerebral cortex. Efferent or *corticofugal* fibers originate in many regions of the cerebral cortex and descend to the basal ganglia, diencephalon, brain stem nuclei, and spinal cord.

Several of the more prominent fasciculi within the subcortical white matter will now be described, as they are exposed in the process of dissection. The **right hemisphere** has already been sectioned to a level above 1.5 cm above the corpus callosum (see Fig. 6-9). This leaves the cingulate gyrus of the hemisphere intact. Identify the cingulate gyrus which encircles the corpus callosum. The *cingulum*, which is the association bundle of the limbic lobe, lies immediately beneath the cortex of this gyrus on the medial aspect of the hemisphere and follows its C-shaped course.

The cingulum is exposed by dissection in an anteroposterior direction with the blunt end of the scalpel. The objective is to remove the cortex of the cingulate gyrus for a distance of 6–7 cm midway between the occipital and frontal poles. Students should examine the coronal section of the brain (Figs. 13-14 and 13-17) and locate the cingulum before attempting the dissection. Once the thin layer of cortex has been removed, the cingulum may be transected in its midregion with the blade of the scalpel. Grasp one end of the transected cingulum with forceps and tear it forward. The course of the cingulum and its fibrous nature will be seen readily. The same procedure may be followed with the other end of the transected cingulum. A similar dissection of the intact cingulate gyrus of the opposite hemisphere will expose the left cingulum as well (Fig. 7-1). Note that

Figure 7-1. Dissection of the right cerebral hemisphere to demonstrate some of the long association bundles of the subcortical white matter: the arcuate fasciculus, the superior longitudinal fasciculus, and the cingulum.

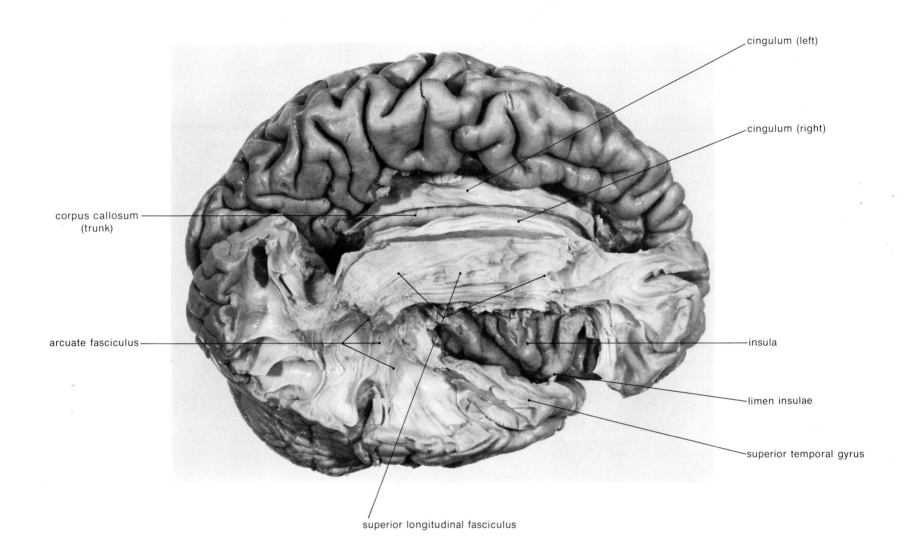

cingulum (left)

cingulum (right)

corpus callosum
(trunk)

arcuate fasciculus

insula

limen insulae

superior temporal gyrus

superior longitudinal fasciculus

49

these prominent association fasciculi are located on each side of the midline and that their constituent fibers run at right angle to those of the underlying corpus callosum. They connect various cortical areas of the frontal and parietal lobes with the temporal lobe of the same hemisphere.

Short association fibers may be demonstrated by inserting the blunt end of the scalpel handle into any of the remaining intact gyri from the **right hemisphere** to a depth of not more than 5 mm. Carefully pry up a piece of the cortex with the scalpel and notice the fibrous texture of the underlying white matter arching around the floor of the sulcus (see Fig. 1-1). Note also that the orientation of the short association fibers is perpendicular to the long axis of the gyri they interconnect.

The *superior longitudinal fasciculus* may now be disclosed beneath the lateral convex surface of the right hemisphere. The opercular cortex of the frontal and parietal lobes has already been removed to uncover the insula. Dissecting in a rostrocaudal direction from above the midpoint of the insula, remove the remaining cortex on the dorsolateral surface of the frontal and parietal lobes (Figs. 7-1 and 7-2). Extend the dissection toward both the frontal and the occipital poles. The superior longitudinal fasciculus is most compact and therefore easiest to demonstrate in its midportion above the insula. From this point its fibers radiate to the parietal and occipital cortices. Many fibers of this association bundle arch around the posterior end of the lateral sulcus to enter the temporal lobe as well. Because of its curved course, this component of the superior longitudinal fasciculus is called the *arcuate fasciculus*.

Now carefully remove the cortex of the insula by blunt dissection in a radial manner, beginning at the limen insulae. Before proceeding with the dissection, examine the brain sections shown in Figs. 13-14, 13-15, 13-54, and 13-55, to gain an appreciation of the size and layered arrangement of the structures beneath the insular cortex.

Immediately beneath the cortex you will notice a thin layer of fibers thrown into ridges that correspond to the gyri of the insula. This is the *extreme capsule;* it is very thin and easily missed if more than just the cortical layer is removed. The components of the extreme capsule include short association fibers of the insular cortex and of the cortex of the frontal, parietal, and temporal opercula. Beneath the extreme capsule is a thin layer of gray matter called the *claustrum,* the functions and connections of which are not well known.

This is also a thin sheet and may be very easily missed in the gross dissection.

Now, by dissecting parallel with the long axis of the temporal lobe, remove the cortex and the superficial white matter on the dorsal and lateral surfaces of the superior temporal gyrus. The middle temporal gyrus may be included as well. Beginning at the limen insulae, remove thin layers (about 0.5–1.0 mm thick) of the subcortical white matter. These layers may be stripped backward along the temporal lobe where the fibers appear to course under those of the arcuate fasciculus. Continue the dissection forward around the stem of the lateral sulcus into the frontal lobe. This procedure exposes the *inferior occipitofrontal fasciculus* (Fig. 7-2). Remove the arcuate fasciculus by making a shallow incision across its main trunk as it curves ventrally from the parietal lobe into the temporal lobe (Fig. 7-2). Pull away the temporal portion of this fasciculus. You may now follow the course of the fibers of the inferior occipitofrontal fasciculus to the occipital lobe. Lying ventral to and in intimate relation with the inferior occipitofrontal fasciculus is the *uncinate fasciculus* (Fig. 7-2), which curves sharply around the stem of the lateral sulcus. The uncinate fasciculus interconnects the orbital and the middle and inferior frontal gyri with the anterior temporal lobe cortex.

Removal of the claustrum will now expose the *external capsule,* which is a thin lamina of white matter that overlies the lateral border of the lenticular (lentiform) nucleus (Fig. 7-2). It is a component of the projection fiber system of the cerebrum, conveying fibers from the cerebral cortex to the putamen and the reticular formation of the brain stem. Remove this sheet of white matter by inserting the spatula into the capsule (to a depth not exceeding 1 mm) just above the inferior occipitofrontal fasciculus. Lift a small flap of fibers upward toward the superior longitudinal fasciculus (see Fig. 1-2). This ensures that the strip will tear along natural cleavage planes and disclose the fibrous nature of the capsule. The fibers will appear to terminate at the *circular sulcus* of the insula, perpendicular to those of the superior longitudinal fasciculus. In fact they do not; rather, they continue under this bundle as will be seen shortly.

Continue the dissection until the outer surface of the *putamen* is

Figure 7-2. Dissection of the right cerebral hemisphere to demonstate the external capsule, the inferior longitudinal fasciculus, and the uncinate fasciculus.

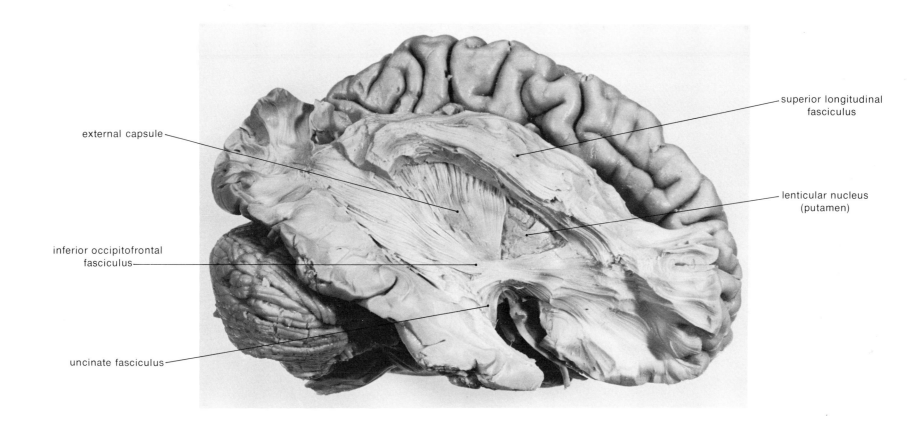

external capsule

superior longitudinal
fasciculus

lenticular nucleus
(putamen)

inferior occipitofrontal
fasciculus

uncinate fasciculus

reached. This nucleus is easily distinguished from the external capsule by its darker color, indicative of its cellular rather than fibrous nature (Figs. 7-2 and 7-3). Note the several *lateral striate arteries* overlying and penetrating the surface of the putamen. These are branches of the anterolateral group of central arteries that arise from the middle cerebral artery as described in Chapter 5.

Remove what remains of the superior longitudinal fasciculus by blunt dissection with the scalpel handle in a radial direction. Remove the inferior occipitofrontal fasciculus as well. You may accomplish this by inserting the spatula underneath the inferior occipitofrontal fasciculus, where it is most compact in the region of the limen insulae, and then stripping it forward toward the frontal pole and backward toward the occipital pole. These procedures expose the *corona radiata*, a radiating crown of fibers that at this stage of the dissection appears to radiate from the upper peripheral border of the putamen out to the frontal, parietal, and temporal lobes in an incomplete circle (Fig. 7-3). Take particular note of those fibers that emerge below the putamen, course through the white matter of the temporal lobe, and then curve backward into the occipital lobe. These make up the *geniculocalcarine tract*, which arises from neurons of the lateral geniculate nucleus of the thalamus, curves laterally beneath the lenticular nucleus, and ultimately terminates in the visual cortex (Fig. 7-3). In so doing, this tract forms a loop (Meyer's loop) within the medullary center of the temporal lobe. It is for this reason that tumors of the temporal lobe or occlusion of temporal branches of the middle cerebral artery may result in homonymous visual field defects.

The large nuclear mass located near the inferior surface of the hemisphere, referred to collectively as the *corpus striatum*, is composed the the *lenticular nucleus* and the *caudate nucleus*. The lenticular nucleus consists of two nuclei; the more medial is the *globus pallidus*, the more lateral is the *putamen* (Figs. 13-16, 13-17, 13-18, 13-39, 13-54). With the external capsule of the right hemisphere already removed, the lateral surface of the putamen should now be fully exposed. Follow the putamen to the base of the hemisphere and demonstrate by careful dissection around the bottom of the anterior limb of the internal capsule its continuity with the head of the caudate nucleus, which lies medial to the anterior limb of the internal capsule (Fig. 7-4). Carefully shell out the putamen by blunt dissection in a radial direction to reveal the lighter colored and more fibrous

globus pallidus. The line of separation between these two nuclei will not be as sharp as it appears in sections of the brain (see external medullary lamina in Fig. 13-17). Now remove the globus pallidus in the same way. This exposes the lateral aspect of the internal capsule (Fig. 7-5).

The internal capsule is a compact band of fibers at the base of the hemisphere formed by the covergence of the corona radiata. The internal capsule is the largest and perhaps the most important component of the projection fiber system of the cerebrum. In horizontal section, the internal capsule is shaped like an open V, with the apex of the V directed medially. The apex of the V corresponds to the *genu of the internal capsule*. In front of the genu is the *anterior limb*, and behind it is the *posterior limb of the internal capsule* (see Figs. 13-37, 13-38, and 13-39). Students are well advised to review at this time the origins and terminations of the various fiber components of the internal capsule. Since corticipetal and corticofugal projection fibers are concentrated in the internal capsule, hemorrhage or occlusion of the lateral striate arteries or the anterior choroidal artery, which together supply most of the internal capsule, results in widespread sensory and motor deficits.

The large neocortical commissure, the *corpus callosum*, has already been seen in the floor of the longitudinal cerebral fissure. For an aid to defining the parts of the corpus callosum, refer to the sagittal section of the brain shown in Figure 6-3 and Figure 13-1. The commissural fibers in the midregion constitute the *trunk of the corpus callosum*. Note that the corpus callosum is shorter than the hemisphere. Its posterior end is thickened and, as the *splenium of the corpus callosum*, accommodates fibers interconnecting the cortices of the occipital lobe. The somewhat smaller anterior end, the *genu of the corpus callosum*, contains fibers interconnecting the frontal lobe cortices. The thin shelf of fibers projecting downward and backward from the genu is the *rostrum of the corpus callosum*. The rostrum is continuous with the *lamina terminalis*, which will be identified at a later stage of the dissection.

Upon entering the medullary center, the laterally directed fibers of the corpus callosum fan out to all parts of the cortex as the *radiations of the corpus callosum*. Remove the cortex on the medial surface of both right and left hemispheres by dissection in an anteroposterior direction for a depth of about 1 cm. This procedure removes the medial frontal gyrus, the paracentral lobule, and the precuneus. The

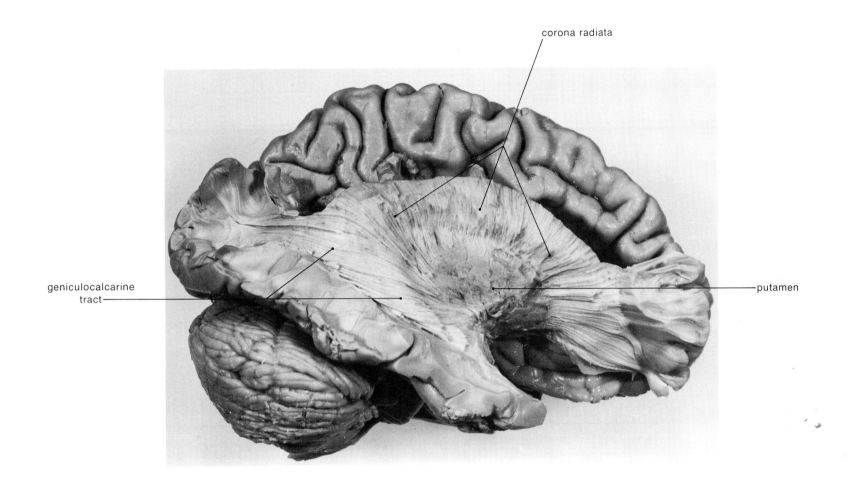

corona radiata

geniculocalcarine
tract

putamen

Figure 7-3. Dissection of the right cerebral hemisphere to demonstrate the projection fibers of the corona radiata and the location of the putamen.

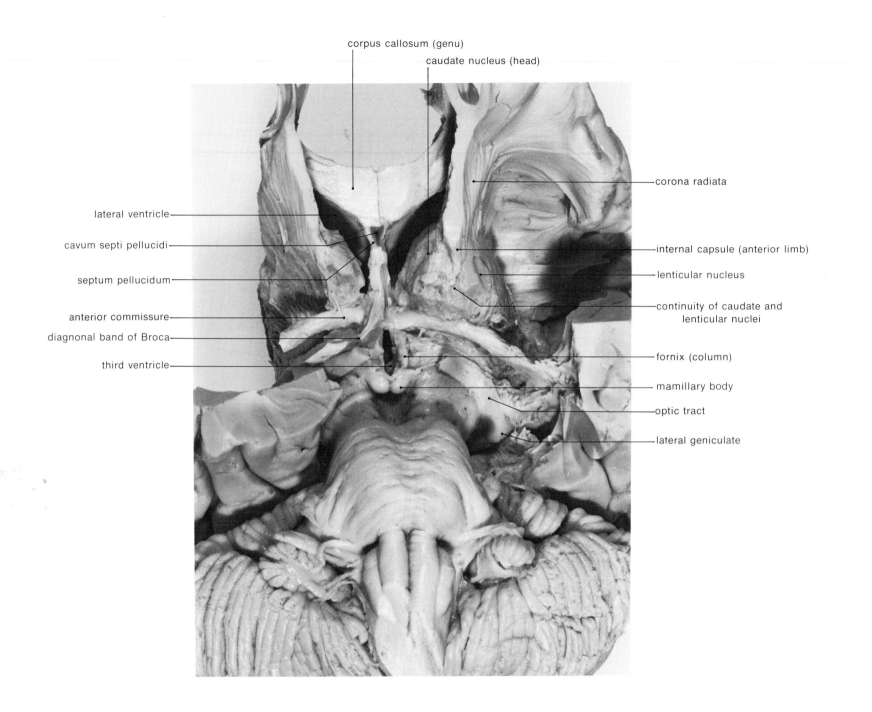

corpus callosum (genu)

caudate nucleus (head)

corona radiata

lateral ventricle

cavum septi pellucidi

septum pellucidum

internal capsule (anterior limb)

lenticular nucleus

continuity of caudate and
lenticular nuclei

anterior commissure

diagnonal band of Broca

fornix (column)

third ventricle

mamillary body

optic tract

lateral geniculate

54

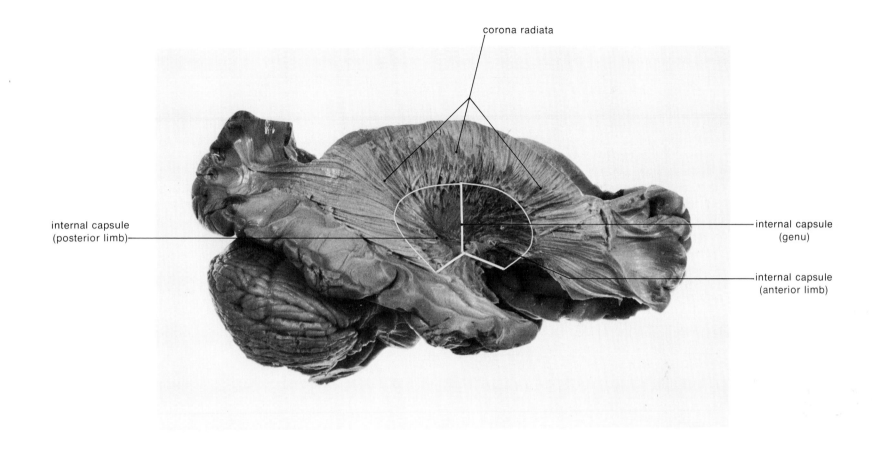

corona radiata

internal capsule
(posterior limb)

internal capsule
(genu)

internal capsule
(anterior limb)

Figure 7-4. Dissection of the inferior portion of the frontal lobe to demonstrate the continuity of the caudate nucleus with the putamen around the anterior limb of the internal capsule, the course of the anterior commissure, and the diagonal band of Broca.

Figure 7-5. Dissection of the right cerebral hemisphere to demonstrate the continuity of the corona radiata with the internal capsule by removal of the lenticular nucleus. The solid white line demonstrates the location of the three named parts of the internal capsule.

cingula are removed in the process as well. The radiations of the corpus callosum may now be seen spreading laterally into each hemisphere, interconnecting vast neopallial areas of the cortex (Fig. 7-6). At the rostral end, the commissural fibers of the genu sweep in a pincer movement toward the frontal poles. The resulting U-shaped configuration is called the *frontal forceps*. A similar but larger sweep of fibers into the occipital pole is called the *occipital forceps*.

The forceps can be better visualized if you scoop out the cortex of the medial surface of the frontal lobe in front of the genu and of the parietal and occipital lobes immediately behind the splenium (Fig. 7-6). There are several other smaller commissures of the brain; these will be identified later in the dissection and include the anterior, hippocampal, habenular, and posterior commissures, as well as commissures of the superior and inferior colliculi.

One remaining component of the corpus striatum yet to be seen is the *caudate nucleus*. The caudate nucleus lies medial to the internal capsule. It can be exposed by cutting away part of the corpus callosum. To accomplish this, make two longitudinal incisions in the trunk of the corpus callosum extending from the splenium to the genu on the **right side only.** The first of these is made with the

blade of the scalpel slightly to the right of the midline. This should be sufficiently deep to just enter the lateral ventricle. The second and parallel incision is made approximately 1.5 cm lateral to the first one and should lie just medial to the corona radiata. Join these incisions by horizontal cuts through both the genu and the splenium of the corpus callosum and lift out that portion of the trunk of the corpus callosum thus incised. This uncovers the right lateral ventricle. The enlarged *head of the caudate nucleus* may be seen lying along the medial surface of the anterior limb of the internal capsule and bulging into the ventricle. The tail of the caudate nucleus extends backward from the head along the lateral edge of the ventricle and enters the temporal lobe. The position of the caudate nucleus in relation to the lateral ventricle medially and the corona radiata laterally is shown clearly in Figs. 9-2 and 9-3.

The anatomic relationships of the many structures identified thus far (insula, extreme capsule, claustrum, external capsule, putamen, globus pallidus, internal capsule, caudate nucleus, and lateral ventricle) should now be reviewed by examining the horizontal and coronal brain sections shown in Figures 13-16, 13-17, 13-18, 13-39, and 13-54.

Figure 7-6. Dorsal view of a dissection of the hemispheres to show the relation of the radiations of the corpus callosum to the corona radiata along with the frontal and occipital forceps.

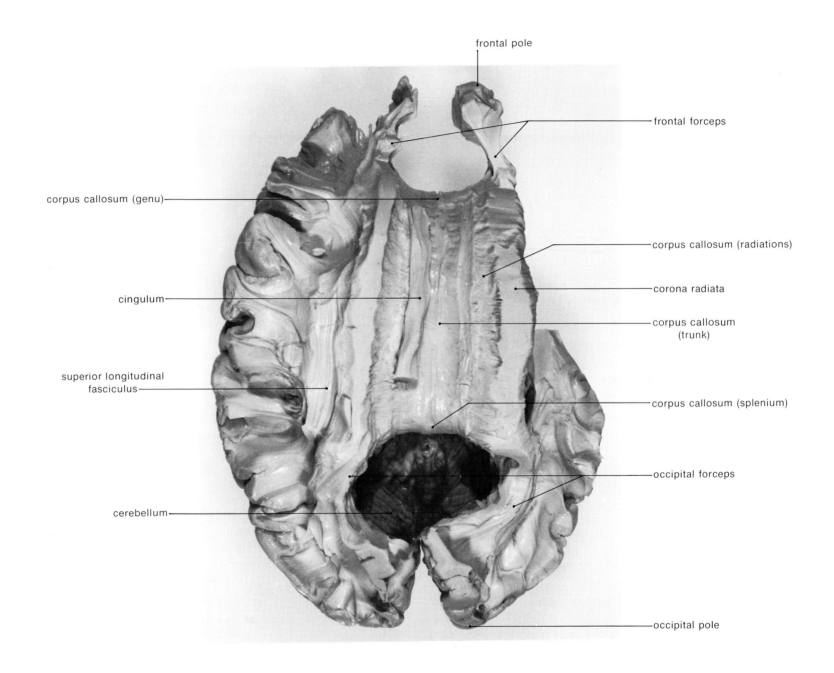

frontal pole

frontal forceps

corpus callosum (genu)

corpus callosum (radiations)

corona radiata

cingulum

corpus callosum (trunk)

superior longitudinal fasciculus

corpus callosum (splenium)

occipital forceps

cerebellum

occipital pole

8

Lateral Cerebral Ventricle and Rhinencephalon

Lateral Cerebral Ventricle

The brain is not a solid structure. Rather, it encloses a series of communicating cavities, which in life are filled with cerebrospinal fluid. These central cavities, called *ventricles*, are four in number: the paired *lateral ventricles* (representing the first two ventricles), located deep within the substance of the cerebral hemispheres; the *third ventricle*, which is a slitlike vertical cavity in the midline between the two halves of the diencephalon; and the *fourth ventricle*, a rhomboid-shaped cavity located within the pons and the medulla.

The unusual but characteristic C shape of the lateral ventricles in the adult brain has its origin in the embryologic development of the telencephalon. In the human embryo of about 35 days (9mm), five secondary brain vesicles may be identified. The cavities within these vesicles are the primitive ventricles. The rostral-most telencephalon at this stage consists of two lateral evaginations surrounding the primitive lateral ventricles, which are in wide communication with the cavity of the diencephalon, the future third ventricle. The primitive cortex of the telencephalon ultimately develops into the massive cerebral hemispheres. This is accomplished by rapid growth forward, upward, and then backward and to a lesser extent downward, overgrowing the diencephalon, the mesencephalon, and part of the metencephalon. In this manner the cerebral hemispheres assume a roughly horseshoe-shaped configuration by the time the fetus is 6 months old.

In the course of its growth, the telencephalic cortex takes with it several associated structures, including the central cavities, which are destined to become the paired lateral ventricles of the adult brain. Hence, the ventricles also assume a C-shaped configuration deep within the hemispheres. Students are advised to examine the photograph of the cast of the cerebral ventricles shown in Figure 8-1 before exposing them in the brain specimen.

The trunk of the corpus callosum, which forms the roof of the ventricle, has been removed from the right hemisphere of the specimen in the previous chapter. Looking down into the cavity of the ventricle reveals the *frontal horn* and the *central part* or *body of the lateral ventricle*. The frontal horn projects forward into the frontal lobe. The rostral curvature of the frontal horn is produced by the overlying genu and the rostrum of the corpus callosum. The vertical medial wall is composed of a thin sheet of gray and white matter known as the *septum pellucidum* (Figs. 6-3, 13-15, 13-16, 13-37, and 13-38). Touch the septum pellucidum with a finger or a blunt probe and notice how thin it is. The frontal horns of the lateral ventricles lie on each side of it. The septum pellucidum is, in reality, two membranes with a narrow vertical cavity between them—the *cavum septi pellucidi* (see Fig. 7-4). This cavity, however, does not normally communicate with the cavity of the ventricles. The enlarged head of the

Figure 8-1. Cast of the ventricles of the brain. In order to support the weight of the fourth ventricle in this cast, the cerebral aqueduct was made larger than it is in the living brain.

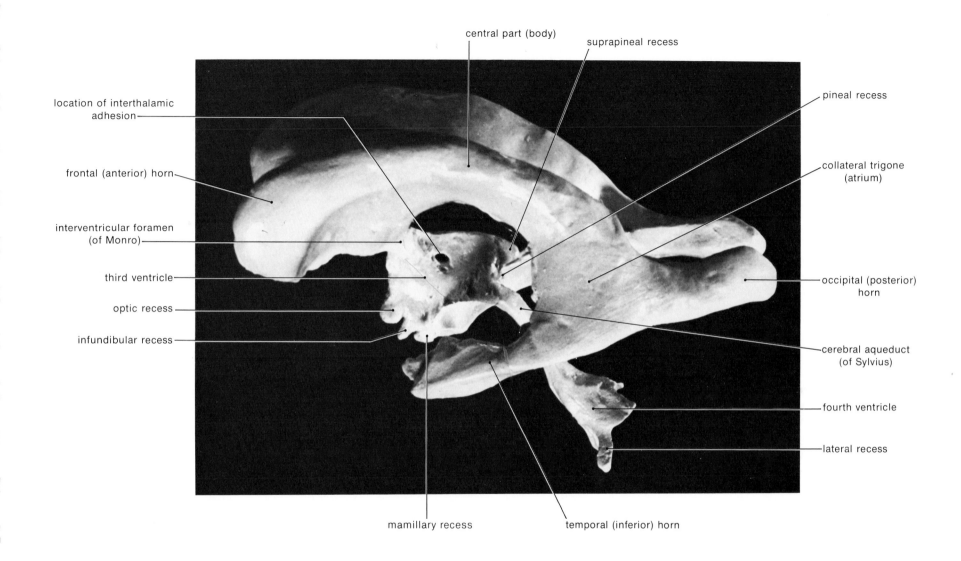

central part (body)

suprapineal recess

location of interthalamic adhesion

pineal recess

frontal (anterior) horn

collateral trigone (atrium)

interventricular foramen (of Monro)

third ventricle

occipital (posterior) horn

optic recess

infundibular recess

cerebral aqueduct (of Sylvius)

fourth ventricle

lateral recess

mamillary recess

temporal (inferior) horn

caudate nucleus, lying medial to the anterior limb of the internal capsule and bulging into the ventricle, forms the floor and the lateral wall of the frontal horn. The inferior surface of the trunk of the corpus callosum forms its roof. Situated on the medial side of the floor of the ventricle about 2.5 cm from the rostral tip of the frontal horn is the *interventricular foramen* (of Monro). This is a narrow communicating channel between the right and left lateral ventricles and the third ventricle located in the midline of the diencephalon. Follow the choroid plexus of the right lateral ventricle forward to the point at which it appears to terminate. Insert a probe into the opening just anterior to this point; this is the interventricular foramen. Note that the interventricular foramen marks the junction between the frontal horn and the central part of the lateral ventricle.

At about the level of the interventricular foramen the caudate nucleus begins to taper into a tail that occupies the lateral wall of the central part of the lateral ventricle. Notice three or four veins traversing the ventricular surface of the caudate nucleus. These are the *transverse caudate veins*. They drain into the *thalamostriate* or *terminal vein*, which lies in a shallow groove where the tail of the caudate nucleus and the superior surface of the thalamus meet. This groove is known as the *terminal sulcus* (see Fig. 9-2). At the level of the interventricular foramen, the thalamostriate vein is joined by the *choroidal vein* to form the *internal cerebral vein*. Both the right and left internal cerebral veins pass backward in the tela choroidea along the dorsomedian surface of the thalamus and then unite beneath the splenium to form the *great cerebral vein* (of Galen). You will not be able to see these latter two veins yet in the dissection.

Running alongside the terminal vein is a thin bundle of fibers known as the *stria terminalis* (see Fig. 9-3). This band of fibers originates from neurons in the amygdaloid nuclei of the temporal lobe, follows the curvature of the tail of the caudate nucleus, and then curves ventrally at the level of the interventricular foramen to terminate in the *septal area* and the preoptic, ventromedial, and anterior hypothalamic nuclei. Some of its fibers, however, join the *stria medullaris thalami;* others across the midline, enter the stria terminalis of the opposite side, and end in the contralateral amygdaloid nucleus.

Most of the medial floor of the central part of the lateral ventricle is formed by the superior surface of the thalamus. Lying on this surface is an evagination of highly vascular pia mater enveloped by choroidal epithelial cells. This is the *choroid plexus* of the lateral ventricle, which together with similar plexuses in the third and fourth ventricles is responsible for the production of cerebrospinal fluid. Immediately under the corpus callosum and contained within the medial walls of this portion of the lateral ventricle is the body of the fornix—a projection fiber bundle of the hippocampal formation, which will be described in detail later in the dissection.

The *temporal horn of the lateral ventricle* in the **right hemisphere** may now be exposed. With the blade of a scalpel, transect the projection fibers of the corona radiata as they emerge from the posterior limb of the internal capsule. Begin near the genu of the internal capsule and then curve backward, downward, and forward into the white matter of the temporal lobe. The incision should stop a few centimeters short of the temporal pole, and it should be just deep enough to enter the cavity of the temporal horn without damaging the structures within it. Reflect the flap of white matter so that the cavity of the ventricle is now visible and remove enough of this overlying white matter to expose the entire temporal horn. Remove the white matter extending into the occipital lobe as well to expose the *occipital horn of the lateral ventricle* (Fig. 8-2). This procedure removes some of the fibers of the geniculocalcarine tract, described in Chapter 7.

The shape and size of the occipital horn are variable. In some specimens the occipital horn may be obliterated or represented as a short, caudally directed diverticulum, whereas in others it may extend for some distance into the occipital lobe. At the junction of the body with the temporal and occipital horns, the ventricle assumes an expanded triangular shape known as the *collateral trigone* (atrium) (see Fig. 8-2). Within the medial wall of the occipital horn and the trigone, two longitudinally directed eminences can be seen. The more dorsal of these, the *bulb of the occipital horn*, is caused by the callosal fibers of the forceps major curving backward and encroaching on the medial surface of the occipital horn. The more ventral and the more prominent of the two is called the *calcar avis*. It is caused by association fibers beneath the deep calcarine sulcus indenting the medial wall of the ventricle.

Figure 8-2. Dissection of the right cerebral hemisphere to expose the central part and the occipital and temporal horns of the lateral cerebral ventricle.

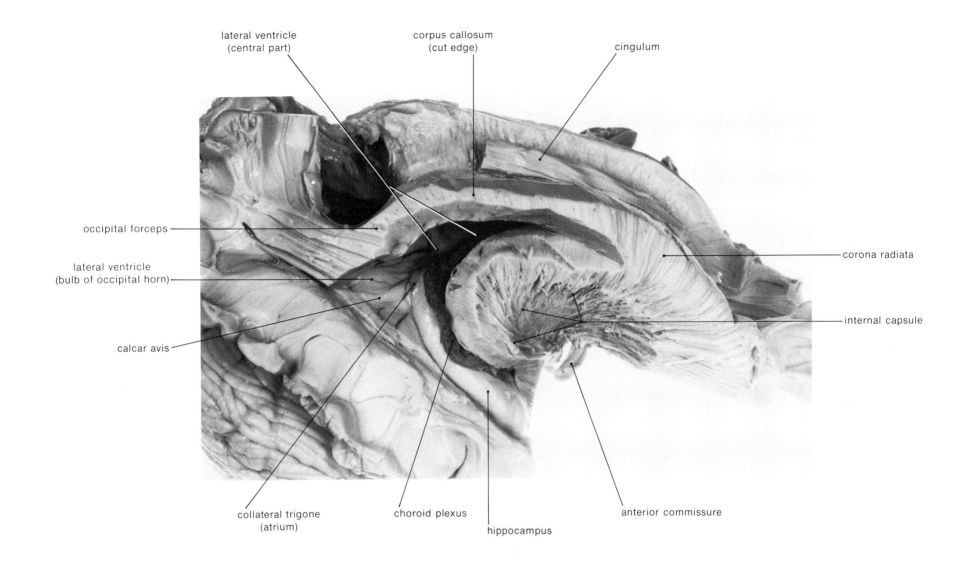

lateral ventricle
(central part)

corpus callosum
(cut edge)

cingulum

occipital forceps

lateral ventricle
(bulb of occipital horn)

calcar avis

corona radiata

internal capsule

collateral trigone
(atrium)

choroid plexus

hippocampus

anterior commissure

61

A very prominent inverted gyrus occupies most of the floor and the medial wall of the temporal horn. This is the *hippocampus* (Figs. 8-2, 8-3, 13-19, and 13-40). It is sometimes easier to visualize the hippocampus as a gyrus that has rolled itself in tightly around the lips of the *hippocampal sulcus,* found on the medial surface of the temporal lobe (see Figs. 8-3 and 13-40). This inwardly bulging gyrus thus forms the eminence seen throughout the length of the temporal horn of the lateral ventricle.

Much of the hippocampus may be obscured by the overlying choroid plexus. With forceps, strip away the choroid plexus, noting its attachment along the *choroidal fissure.* The anterior expanded end of the hippocampus is grooved, giving it the appearance of a foot and hence the name *pes hippocampi* for this region (Figs. 8-3 and 13-41).

Beneath the ependyma and covering the ventricular surface of the hippocampus is a thin layer of efferent fibers known as the *alveus* (Fig. 13-17). These fibers arise mainly from the pyramidal cells of the hippocampal cortex. They converge near the medial border of the hippocampus to form a fringe of fibers known as the *fimbria* of the hippocampus (Fig. 8-3). The fimbria courses backward following the hippocampus. Beneath the splenium of the corpus callosum it arches forward over the thalamus, forming the *crus* of the fornix. In the following chapter we will see how both the right and left crura converge in the median plane beneath the trunk of the corpus callosum to form the *body* of the fornix.

As the cerebral hemispheres and the corpus callosum expand dorsally and laterally over the diencephalon during fetal development, they bring with them their pial investment. In so doing, a double layer of vascular pia mater is formed that comes to occupy the transverse fissure and is referred to as the *tela choroidea.* Evagination along the choroidal fissure gives rise to the choroid plexuses of the lateral ventricles. The tela choroidea of the transverse fissure is also continuous with and gives rise to the choroid plexus of the third ventricle (yet to be examined) by evaginating into this ventricle along its narrow roof. In addition to the tela choroidea, the internal cerebral veins, branches of the posterior cerebral artery, and arteries to the choroid plexus of the third and lateral ventricles occupy the transverse cerebral fissure. The transverse cerebral fissure will be described in more detail in the next chapter.

Rhinencephalon

The term "rhinencephalon" is derived from the Greek meaning olfactory brain or "nose brain." It is not a discrete part of the brain that can be isolated by a simple dissection; rather, it is a complex part of the brain that functionally involves many structures. Classically it is composed of those structures responsible for the primary reception of impulses resulting from olfactory stimuli, including those that in the process of evolution have lost much of their original olfactory function. Although the latter components may still receive secondary olfactory relays, they have become more important in the integration of visceral stimuli with emotional behavioral patterns. In macrosmatic animals (those animals with a highly developed sense of smell), the rhinencephalon is well developed and is essential to the survival of the animal and the species. In microsmatic man (having a less acute sense of smell), however, the rhinencephalon is not as well developed and is of lesser functional importance. This phenomenon is illustrated by the very fact that there are common names for the loss of the senses of vision and of hearing—blindness and deafness, respectively—but none for the loss of the sense of smell. The technical word is *anosmia.* In humans, therefore, the term rhinencephalon is usually and appropriately restricted to those structures, listed below, that receive direct olfactory projections only. The related anatomic areas on the medial surface of the hemisphere that are not primarily olfactory in function are included in the *limbic lobe* and *limbic system* and will be discussed in the following chapter.

Now examine the ventral (inferior) surface of the **left hemisphere,** which should be intact. The *olfactory bulb* and the *olfactory tract* overlie the *olfactory sulcus* on each side of the longitudinal fissure (see Fig. 6-6). Each olfactory bulb receives about 20 olfactory nerve fascicles that consist of a variable number of unmyelinated axons (fila olfactoria) of bipolar cells located in the specialized epithelium of the nasal mucosa. These nerve fascicles enter the cranial cavity by traversing

Figure 8-3. Dissection of the left temporal lobe demonstrating the structures surrounding the hippocampal sulcus. The body and column of the fornix and the mamillary body have been dissected free from the rest of the brain to show their continuity with the hippocampus.

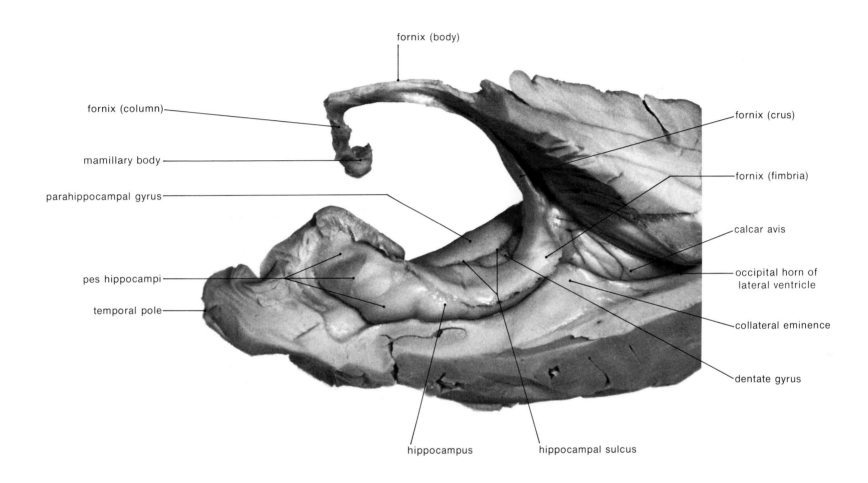

fornix (body)

fornix (column)

fornix (crus)

mamillary body

fornix (fimbria)

parahippocampal gyrus

calcar avis

pes hippocampi

occipital horn of
lateral ventricle

temporal pole

collateral eminence

dentate gyrus

hippocampus

hippocampal sulcus

the cribriform plate of the ethmoid bone (see Fig. 2-2) and synapse with the dendrites of large mitral cells within the olfactory bulb. Axons of the mitral cells pass caudally in the *olfactory tract*. Just in front of the anterior perforated substance and lateral to the optic chiasma the olfactory tract widens into a triangular area known as the *olfactory trigone*.

Classically it is said that three small fiber bundles pass caudally from the region of the olfactory trigone; they have been described as the *medial*, the *intermediate*, and the *lateral olfactory striae*. However, recent studies using more modern tracing techniques have shown that this is no longer tenable. The following represents a more current account of the olfactory brain of man.

A few fibers of the olfactory tract curve medially at the trigone to terminate in the *anterior olfactory nucleus* (Fig. 8-4). It is difficult if at all possible to demonstrate their course past this nucleus. Still fewer fibers continue caudally from the trigone to terminate in the thin layer of cortex of the *anterior perforated substance*. The majority of fibers of the olfactory tract curve laterally from the trigone as the *lateral olfactory stria*. This stria curves sharply again around the limen insulae in the stem of the lateral sulcus toward the medial parts of the temporal lobe. In its course the fibers of the lateral olfactory stria terminate in the following areas: (1) a thin layer of cortex that overlies the stria *(lateral olfactory gyrus)*, (2) the corticomedial division of the *amygdaloid nucleus* of the temporal lobe, (3) the cortex of the *uncus*, and (4) the rostral portion of the *parahippocampal gyrus*. These areas constitute the *primary olfactory cortex* of the human brain (Fig. 8-4). These structures are sometimes referred to as the *piriform lobe* of the brain because of their fancied resemblance to the shape of a pear (from the Latin word "pirum" meaning a pear) in macrosmatic animals. The term *prepiriform cortex* refers to the cortex of the lateral olfactory gyrus as well as the cortex of the limen insulae. The term *entorhinal area* (derived from two Greek words "ento" meaning within and "rhis" meaning nose) is the cortex of the anterior part of the parahippocampal gyrus medial to the rhinal sulcus. These structures may be better seen if the anterior portion of the temporal lobe is rotated laterally around the stem of the lateral sulcus to expose the structures on the medial surface.

As stated earlier, the rhinencephalon is of little importance to humans. However, testing for the sense of smell in the neurologic examination can provide important diagnostic information. Fractures at the base of the skull in the region of the ethmoid bone may shear off the olfactory fila as they penetrate the cribriform plate thus producing bilateral anosmia. Unilateral anosmia is frequently a consequence of certain neoplasms of the frontal lobe, especially meningiomas of the sphenoidal ridge and olfactory groove.

Many secondary olfactory tracts originate from the olfactory areas described previously, and proceed, by complicated and diverse circuitry, to the cortex of the cingulate gyrus, the nuclei of the diencephalon, and the brain stem. Although some of these will be seen in the subsequent dissection of the limbic lobe and diencephalon, students are advised to review these olfactory pathways, the description of which may be found in most neuroanatomy textbooks.

It is now possible to demonstrate another of the commissures of the cerebrum, the *anterior commissure*. This compact bundle interconnects the cortex of the anterior portions of each temporal lobe and such fibers represent the largest component of the anterior commissure. A few olfactory axons cross the midline in the anterior commissure to interconnect the olfactory bulbs and anterior olfactory nuclei of the two hemispheres.

Reflect the optic tracts and the optic chiasma backward. The thin layer of cortex seen with a punctate appearance is the *anterior perforated substance*. It is so called because of the many small arterial twigs of the anterior group of ganglionic arteries that puncture the surface of the brain here. Beginning in the midline remove this thin layer of cortex with a small spatula dissecting from side to side. A few millimeters below the surface you will be able to identify a compact bundle of fibers about 4 mm in diameter crossing the midline. This is the *anterior commissure* (see Fig. 7-4). Extend the dissection laterally into each temporal lobe to reveal the course of the commissure. In doing so, note particularly the relationship of this commissure to the anterior limb of the internal capsule, the head of the caudate nucleus, and the putamen (see Figs. 7-4, 13-16, 13-40, and 13-55).

Figure 8-4. Olfactory structures on the inferior surface of the brain. The anterior portion of the temporal lobe has been removed on the right side to provide a better view of the lateral olfactory stria and the anterior perforated substance.

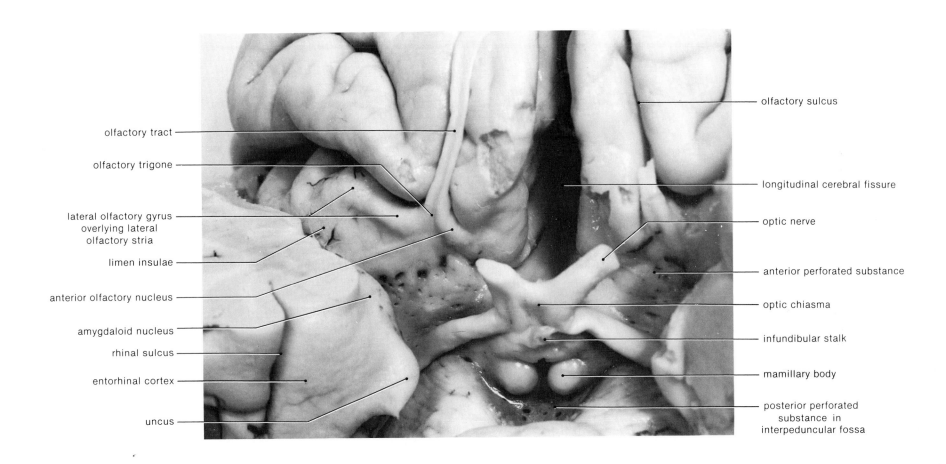

olfactory tract

olfactory trigone

lateral olfactory gyrus
overlying lateral
olfactory stria

limen insulae

anterior olfactory nucleus

amygdaloid nucleus

rhinal sulcus

entorhinal cortex

uncus

olfactory sulcus

longitudinal cerebral fissure

optic nerve

anterior perforated substance

optic chiasma

infundibular stalk

mamillary body

posterior perforated
substance in
interpeduncular fossa

9

Limbic System, Diencephalon, and Third Ventricle

The adjective "limbic" is derived from the Latin word "limbus," meaning a hem or a border. The term was introduced into neuroanatomy in the latter half of the nineteenth century by Pierre Paul Broca to describe those parts of the brain having a highly arched structure that formed a border of cortex and fiber bundles interposed between the neopallium on the one hand and the diencephalon and the brain stem on the other.

The two terms *limbic lobe* and *limbic system* present recurring difficulties for students of neuroanatomy. This is due in part to the lack of uniformity in the terminology used by authors in this field. We have adopted the following definitions, fully realizing that there may be points of argument based on a variety of grounds. The term *limbic lobe* includes the following structures found on the medial surface of the hemisphere: the paraterminal gyrus, the cingulate gyrus, the parahippocampal gyrus, and the narrow strip of cortex lying beneath the splenium of the corpus callosum, the isthmus, or retrosplenial cortex, which joins the cingulate and parahippocampal gyri. The term *limbic system* is a functional more than an anatomic term. Broadly defined, it consists of a number of anatomically distinct but funtionally interrelated structures. The structures implied in the use of this term include all of the components of the limbic lobe plus the hippocampus, dentate gyrus, amygdaloid nuclei, uncus, anterior nucleus of the thalamus, certain nuclei of the hypothalamus, habenular nucleus, interpeduncular nucleus, and nuclei of the midbrain tegmentum. It also includes the following fiber bundles or pathways interconnecting the many nuclei listed above: the fornix, stria terminalis, mamillothalamic tract, medial and lateral longitudinal striae, stria medullaris thalami, medial forebrain bundle, cingulum, and anterior commissure. Functionally, the limbic system serves to integrate autonomic, somatic, and visceral activities related to the preservation of the individual and the species and to the generation and expression of behavior that would appear to be related to emotional states such as fear, anger, and depression. It is also recognized to be important in the phenomenon of recent memory and learning.

In the dissection of this region of the brain, it will be possible to identify most of the anatomic components of the limbic system, but not necessarily in the order in which they are listed above. Two of the cortical components of the limbic lobe (cingulate gyrus and parahippocampal gyrus) were identified in Chapter 6. Review the precise location of these gyri before proceeding further with the dissection.

Examine the superior surface of the **left** half of the corpus callosum, which should still be intact in the brain specimen. If the left cingulum is still present, remove it by tearing it forward to the genu and backward toward the splenium of the corpus callosum. You may now be able to see two small elevated strands of fibers running longitudinally along the dorsal surface of the corpus callosum on the left side. The two on the right side were removed with the corpus callosum previously in order to view the caudate nucleus. These are the *medial* and the *lateral longitudinal striae* (see Fig. 9-1). The more medial is located close to the midline and is smaller than the lateral, which lies 3 to 4 mm more laterally in the callosal sulcus. These striae are regarded as the remnant association fiber bundles of a vestigial gyrus, the *indusium griseum,* which is no longer prominent in the brain of humans. Rather, the indusium griseum in humans is represented by a very thin layer of gray matter that covers the dorsal surface of the corpus callosum. The few fibers of the longitudinal striae continue rostrally around the genu of the corpus callosum to terminate in the cortex of the medial surface of the frontal lobe, and caudally around the splenium of the corpus callosum as part of the *fasciolar gyrus.* The fasciolar gyrus may be seen easily by examining the undersurface of the splenium of the corpus callosum from behind. It is continuous with the dentate gyrus lying in the hippocampal sulcus on the medial surface of the temporal lobe (see Fig. 8-3).

In the brain specimen, the **right** lateral ventricle has been opened to reveal the head and tail of the caudate nucleus in the previous chapter. With the blade of the scalpel, now make a longitudinal incision in the corpus callosum from the genu to the splenium 3–4 mm **left** of the midline. This incision should be of sufficient depth only to enter the lateral ventricle on the left side. The midline portion of the corpus callosum must be preserved. Now with the brain knife remove successive horizontal slices from what remains of the left cerebral hemisphere, starting from the superior surface and working down until the frontal horn and the central part of the left lateral ventricle are exposed. These horizontal slices must terminate medially at the longitudinal incision just made in the left side of the corpus callosum. Both lateral ventricles are now exposed by this procedure, but the midline of the corpus callosum and the structures beneath it are preserved.

Both the right and the left fornices may now be observed from their lateral aspect. Arching upward from the hippocampus, the fibers of the fimbria form the *crus of the fornix,* which is just ventral and lateral to the splenium of the corpus callosum. The two crura of the fornix (one from each side) continue forward over the superior surface of the thalamus and in so doing converge toward the midline. Here they are known as the *body of the fornix,* which lies immediately beneath and attached to the underside of the trunk of the corpus callosum. Just anterior to the interventricular foramina the fornix curves sharply downward as the *columns of the fornix,* which disappear from view. Notice the vertical *septum pellucidum* attached to the corpus callosum above and to the fornix below. With the blade of the scalpel, remove this sickle-shaped septum by cutting along its

attachment to these two structures (see Fig. 9-4 and explanation in legend). Make a horizontal cut with the blade of the scalpel through what remains of the genu and the splenium of the corpus callosum. Lift up the midportion of the corpus callosum, making sure in so doing that it is free from its attachment to the underlying body of the fornix. Care must be taken not to excise the fibers that join the crura of the fornix at the caudal end of the corpus callosum. The fornix may now be viewed from above (Fig. 9-2). At the posterior end of the fornix notice a flat triangular band of fibers joining the crus on the one side with that of the contralateral side. This is the *commissure of the fornix* (hippocampal commissure or psalterium). This is a thin flat commissure adhering closely to the corpus callosum. It may very well have been removed with the corpus callosum.

The *transverse cerebral fissure* may now be identified. It lies in the space above the diencephalon and the midbrain and separates these structures from the cerebral hemispheres above. The tentorium cerebelli lies in the caudal part of the transverse cerebral fissure. Visualizing the precise location of the rostral part of this fissure is a recurring problem for beginning students in neuroanatomy. It is helpful to refer to the embryology of the brain in attempting to describe it. As the cerebral hemispheres and the corpus callosum grow posteriorly over the diencephalon during fetal development they carry with them their pial investment. There is thus formed a double fold of pia with its accompanying vessels, one fold belonging to the telencephalic structures above, and the other belonging to the diencephalic and mesencephalic structures below. The space between the two layers is the transverse cerebral fissure, while the two layers of pia themselves are referred to as the *tela choroidea.* The two lateral edges of the tela choroidea give rise to the choroid plexus of the lateral ventricles by invaginating into these spaces. The floor of the tela choroidea gives rise to the choroid plexus of the third ventricle (yet to be examined) by invaginating downward into this ventricle along its narrow roof. The rostral part of the transverse cerebral fissure therefore takes the shape of a thin, flat arrowhead with a pointed tip and concave sides. In the specimen, these concave sides are represented by the line of attachment of the body and crura of the fornices to the dorsal surface of the thalamus, that is, the choroidal fissure (Fig. 9-2). The rostral part of the transverse cerebral fissure is accented by the solid black line in Figure 9-3.

The anterior part of this fissure is more difficult to visualize than

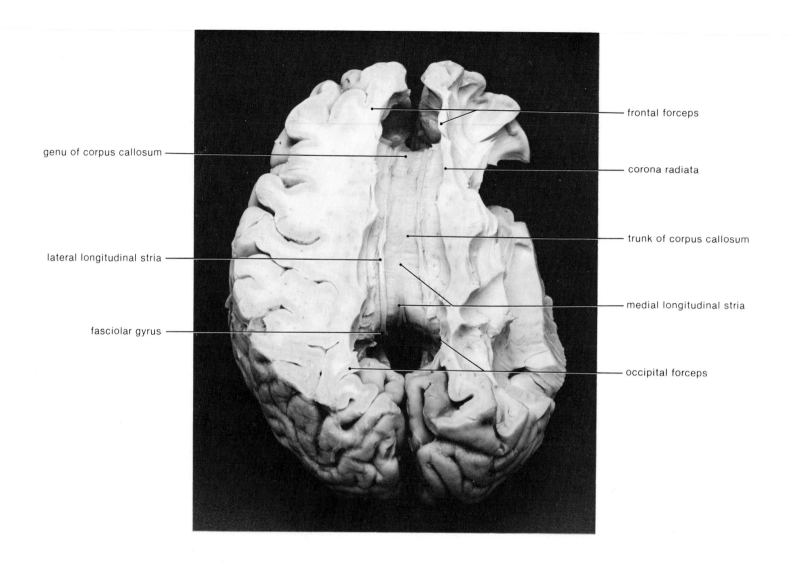

genu of corpus callosum

lateral longitudinal stria

fasciolar gyrus

frontal forceps

corona radiata

trunk of corpus callosum

medial longitudinal stria

occipital forceps

Figure 9-1. View of the dorsal surface of the corpus callosum showing the medial and the lateral longitudinal stria.

68

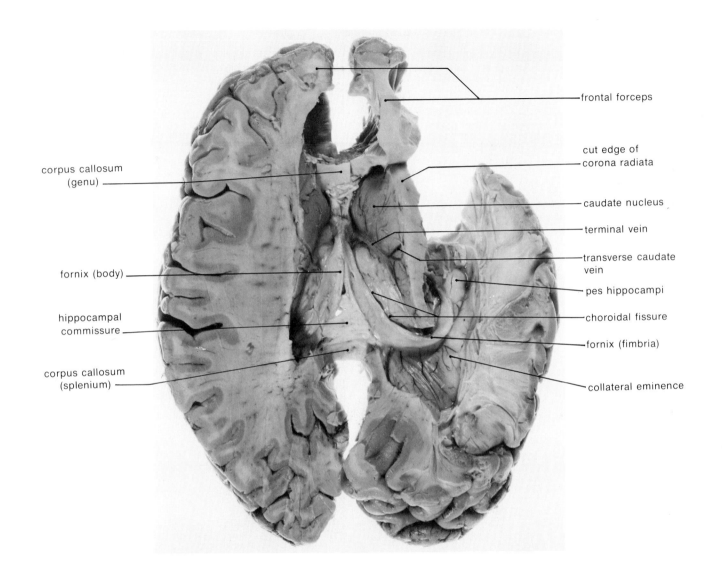

frontal forceps

cut edge of corona radiata

corpus callosum (genu)

caudate nucleus

terminal vein

transverse caudate vein

fornix (body)

pes hippocampi

hippocampal commissure

choroidal fissure

fornix (fimbria)

corpus callosum (splenium)

collateral eminence

Figure 9-2. View of the lateral cerebral ventricles from above. The trunk of the corpus callosum has been removed to show the two crura and bodies of the fornix and the hippocampal commissure.

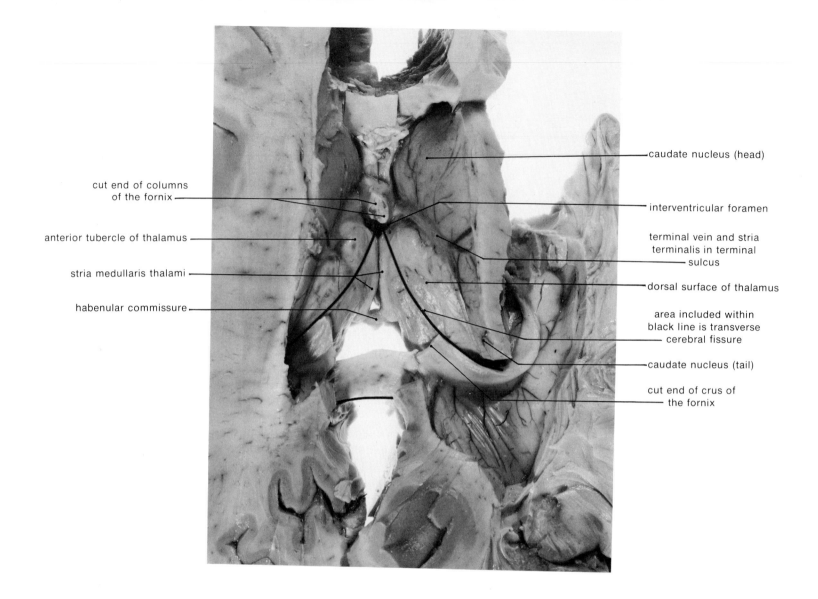

cut end of columns
of the fornix

anterior tubercle of thalamus

stria medullaris thalami

habenular commissure

caudate nucleus (head)

interventricular foramen

terminal vein and stria
terminalis in terminal
sulcus

dorsal surface of thalamus

area included within
black line is transverse
cerebral fissure

caudate nucleus (tail)

cut end of crus of
the fornix

Figure 9-3.   View of the lateral cerebral ventricles and the third ventricle from above. The body of the fornix has been removed by transection of the crura posteriorly and the columns anteriorly at the level of the interventricular foramen. The triangular space included within the solid black lines represents the anterior portion of the transverse cerebral fissure.

it is to demonstrate in the gross specimen. With forceps and scissors remove all of the choroid plexus of the right and left lateral ventricles. Insert a blunt probe into the narrow slit thus produced under the fornix. If the probe is directed laterally, it will emerge through the choroidal fissure of the opposite side. If the probe is directed backward, it will appear beneath the splenium of the corpus callosum. This space is the transverse cerebral fissure.

Cut through the columns of the fornix at the point at which they curve in front of the interventricular foramen and reflect the fornix backward. Remove the body of the fornix and the hippocampal commissure by transecting the two crura (Fig. 9-3). This provides an unobstructed view of the dorsal surface of the thalamus, which is the largest subdivision of the diencephalon. The narrow vertical slit in the midline is the *third ventricle*, which communicates with the lateral ventricles via the interventricular foramen. You may be able to see two narrow folds of choroid plexus hanging down into the ventricle from the tela choroidea and forming the roof of this ventricle. These are quite delicate, however, and may have been torn away upon reflecting the fornix.

The two halves of the thalamus are joined in about 70% of human brains by a small mass of gray matter bridging the third ventricle in the midline. This is the *interthalamic adhesion*. On the dorsomedial surface near the rostral limit of the thalamus notice two small swellings, one on each side; these are the *anterior tubercles of the thalamus*, produced by the underlying *anterior thalamic nuclei* (Fig. 9-3).

Free what remains of the right temproal lobe from the rest of the brain by cutting in the region of the splenium and the limen insulae. This procedure exposes the posterior end of the thalamus, which is composed of a broad cushion-like mass of gray matter known as the *pulvinar*. Beneath the pulvinar are two small elevations in the surface contour. The more medial elevation is the *medial geniculate body*, produced by the underlying *medial geniculate nucleus*. It is a nucleus in the central auditory pathway and receives its afferent connections from the *nucleus of the inferior colliculus* via the *brachium of the inferior colliculus*, both of which will be examined later in the dissection of the brain stem. The axons of the neurons of the medial geniculate nucleus project to the auditory cortex of the temporal lobe via the auditory radiations of the internal capsule.

Just lateral to the medial geniculate body is the *lateral geniculate body*, which marks the location of the *lateral geniculate nucleus*. It is an oval eminence on the posterolateral surface of the thalamus at the termination of the optic tract. This nucleus is associated with the visual pathway; it receives retinal projections from the optic tract and, in turn, projects to the visual cortex above and below the calcarine sulcus. Some fibers of the optic tract bypass the lateral geniculate nucleus, continue in the *brachium of the superior colliculus*, and terminate in the *nucleus of the superior colliculus* and the *pretectal nucleus*. These connections serve as parts of the afferent limb for a variety of motor reflexes that are initiated by visual stimuli, for example, the pupillary light reflex, the accommodation reflex, and reflex movements of the eyes, the eyelids and the head. The superior brachium, which is less obvious than the inferior brachium, passes medially above the medial geniculate body between it and the pulvinar on its way to the superior colliculus. The medial and the lateral geniculate nuclei taken together are sometimes referred to as the *metathalamus*.

Now examine what remains of the right temporal lobe. During fetal development, the hippocampus is formed by a rolling in of the gyrus along a longitudinal sulcus on the medial surface of the temporal lobe. This is the *hippocampal sulcus;* in the adult it becomes almost closed because of the tight rolling of the adjacent cortex. The word "hippocampus" is taken directly from the Greek name for a marine animal, the seahorse. This part of the temporal lobe is so called because of its S-shaped seahorse appearance in cross section. The outer lips of the sulcus are visible on the most medial aspect of the temporal lobe (see Fig. 8-3). Lying in the hippocampal sulcus and immediately adjacent to the fimbria is the *dentate gyrus*, so named because of the serrations on its surface that give it the appearance of many small teeth. The posterior extremity of the dentate gyrus blends into the *fasciolar gyrus*, which curves upward over the splenium of the corpus callosum and is continuous with the indusium griseum. Along its length the hippocampal sulcus separates the dentate gyrus from the *subiculum*, which is the most medial cortex of the parahippocampal gyrus. These three structures—the hippocampus, the dentate gyrus, and the subiculum—are known collectively as the *hippocampal formation*.

The anteromedial portion of the parahippocampal gyrus is curved sharply upon itself to form a hooklike configuration of cortex called the *uncus* (see Fig. 8-4). With the brain knife, make a coronal cut through the hippocampal formation and what remains of the temporal lobe of the right hemisphere. Examine the cut surface and observe again the anatomic arrangement of the structures around the hippocampal sulcus.

The diencephalon is composed of the thalamus, subthalamus, epithalamus, and hypothalamus. The only part of the diencephalon visible on the exterior surface of the brain is the ventral surface of the hypothalamus. Examine the ventral surface of the brain. The hypothalamus is a paired mass of gray matter located on each side of the third ventricle. It is bounded anteriorly by the optic chiasma, posteriorly by the mamillary bodies, and laterally by the optic tracts. A small conical stem emerges from the base of the hypothalamus just behind the optic chiasma in the midline (see Figs. 5-1 and 8-4); it is the *infundibular stalk* (stem) and forms the neural connection between the hypothalamus and the *infundibular process* (posterior pituitary gland) located within the sella turcica. The part of the hypothalamus that is located between the optic chiasma and the mamillary bodies and that produces a bulge on the ventral surface is called the *tuber cinereum* (see Fig. 6-6). The infundibular stalk takes its origin from a thin circular ridge of neural tissue in the midline of the tuber cinereum called the *medium eminence of the hypothalamus*. It is a very small structure, but its size bears no relationship to its importance in the control of the adenohypophysis by the central nervous system. It is here that the hypothalamic-releasing or inhibiting hormones find their way into the pituitary portal vasculature to reach the parenchymal cells of the adenohypophysis.

Now make a midline longitudinal incision through the optic chiasma, the tuber cinereum, and the mamillary bodies. Extend the incision deeper to divide the interthalamic adhesion, the anterior commissure, and the lamina terminalis. The right half of the diencephalon is removed by this procedure, exposing the sagittal surface of the third ventricle and the midline structures of the diencephalon. Direct your attention now to the medial surface of the diencephalon. Identify the *lamina terminalis*, which is an attenuated continuation of the rostrum of the corpus callosum down toward the optic chiasma (Fig. 9-4). This thin lamina represents the anterior limit of the hypothalamus. Near the junction of the lamina terminalis with the rostrum of the corpus callosum, identify the cut surface of the anterior commissure. Just behind it the column of the fornix curves downward into the hypothalamus, forming the anterior wall of the interventricular foramen. Beginning here and extending backward is a

shallow horizontal depression in the wall of the third ventricle; this is the *hypothalamic sulcus*, which represents the line of demarcation between the hypothalamus below and the thalamus above. On the dorsomedial surface of the thalamus, locate a fine ridge of white matter beginning near the anterior tubercle and extending horizontally backward. This is the *stria medullaris thalami*, which is one of the secondary olfactory pathways (Figs. 9-3, 9-4, 9-6, and 9-7). The constituent fibers of the stria medullaris arise from a variety of sources, including the septal area, the hippocampus by way of the fornix, and the amygdaloid nucleus by way of the stria terminalis. The stria medullaris terminates in the habenular nucleus, which forms an enlargement at the end of the tract just at the base of the *pineal gland*. The pineal gland is the conic structure located in the midline above the tectum of the midbrain. Two small commissures are located near the base of the pineal gland. The more dorsal of the two contains fibers of the stria medullaris thalami crossing to the contralateral habenular nucleus. It is called the *habenular commissure* (Figs. 9-3 and 9-5). The more ventral is the *posterior commissure*, lying just above the entrance to the cerebral aqueduct of the midbrain (Fig. 9-4). The stria medullaris thalami, the habenular nuclei and commissure, the posterior commissure, and the pineal gland are referred to collectively as the *epithalamus*.

The cavity of the third ventricle has four small diverticula, called recesses, which are formed by the configuration of the surrounding diencephalic structures (Fig. 9-4 and the cast of the third ventricle in Fig. 8-1).

1. The *optic recess* is located immediately above the optic chiasma, between it and the lamina terminalis.

2. The *infundibular recess* is a funnel-shaped recess projecting into the infundibular stalk.

3. The *pineal recess* projects into the stalk of the pineal gland. It is bounded above by the habenular commissure and below by the posterior commissure.

Figure 9-4. Medial view of the right half of a hemisected brain showing the relationship of diencephalic structures to the cerebral hemisphere and the brain stem. The septum pellucidum has been removed by cutting along its attachment with the corpus callosum and the body of the fornix. The dark cavity just left of center is the frontal horn of the right lateral ventricle.

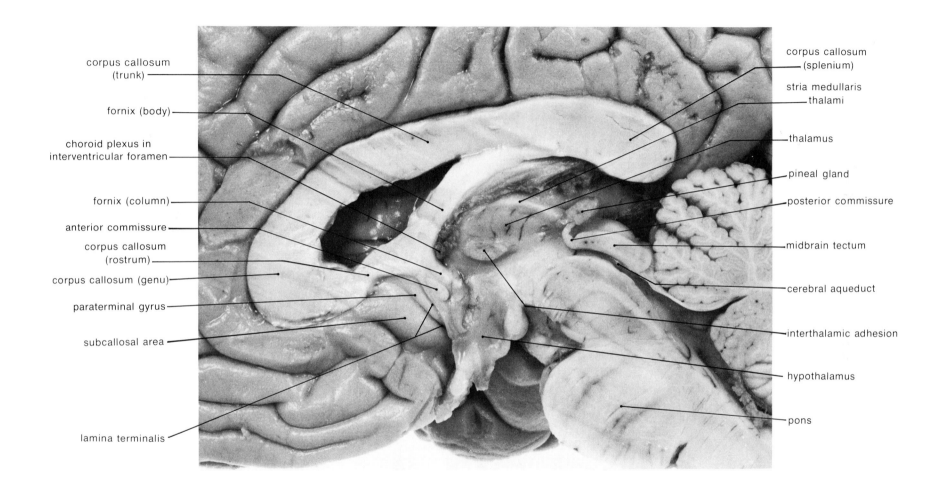

corpus callosum (trunk)

fornix (body)

choroid plexus in interventricular foramen

fornix (column)

anterior commissure

corpus callosum (rostrum)

corpus callosum (genu)

paraterminal gyrus

subcallosal area

lamina terminalis

corpus callosum (splenium)

stria medullaris thalami

thalamus

pineal gland

posterior commissure

midbrain tectum

cerebral aqueduct

interthalamic adhesion

hypothalamus

pons

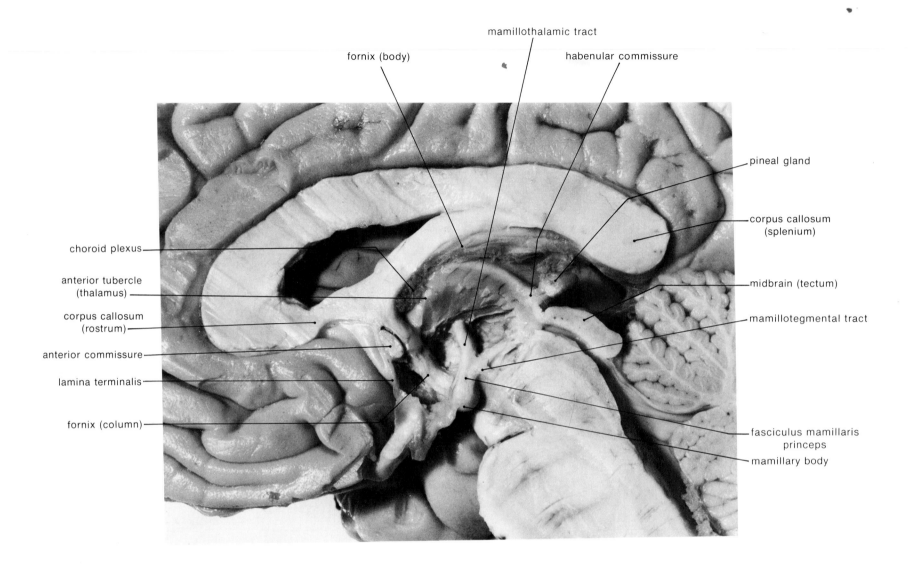

mamillothalamic tract

fornix (body)

habenular commissure

pineal gland

corpus callosum
(splenium)

choroid plexus

anterior tubercle
(thalamus)

corpus callosum
(rostrum)

anterior commissure

lamina terminalis

fornix (column)

midbrain (tectum)

mamillotegmental tract

fasciculus mamillaris
princeps

mamillary body

4. The *suprapineal recess* is a diverticulum of the ventricle located directly above the pineal gland.

The walls of the posterior portion of the third ventricle converge at the junction of the diencephalon with the mesencephalon to form the narrow *cerebral aqueduct* (of Sylvius) traversing the midbrain (Fig. 9-4; see also Fig. 8-1).

The hypothalamus is not only a mass of gray matter; it contains several important fiber bundles, including the dorsal longitudinal fasciculus, the medial forebrain bundle, the fornix, the mamillothalamic tract, and the mamillotegmental tract. It is possible to demonstrate some of the larger and more compact of these bundles. Recall that the columns of the fornix curve ventrally just behind the anterior commissure to distribute their fibers largely, but not exclusively, to the mamillary nuclei of the hypothalamus. Examine the relationship of the fornix column, the mamillothalamic tract, and the mamillotegmental tract to the surrounding hypothalamic tissue shown in Figure 9-5 before attempting the dissection. The column of the fornix may be exposed by carefully removing the hypothalamic tissue surrounding it. This can be accomplished only by dissecting with the small spatula parallel to the long axis of the column. Notice its termination in the mamillary body. In the same manner, the *mamillothalamic tract* can be traced for some distance into the deeper portions of the thalamus. This bundle terminates largely within the anterior nuclear complex of the thalamus. A short distance from its origin, a large branch of the mamillothalamic tract curves caudally as the *mamillotegmental tract* to terminate in the dorsal and ventral tegmental nuclei and the reticular formation of the midbrain.

The final subdivision of the diencephalon, the *subthalamus,* is a region that is not amenable to gross dissection. It lies medial to the internal capsule, ventral to the thalamus, and dorsolateral to the hypothalamus. This area contains several nuclei and fiber tracts related to motor functions. They are the *subthalamic nucleus*, the *zona incerta*, the *lenticular fasciculus*, the *thalamic fasciculus*, and the *subthalamic fasciculus*. These structures are best seen in the coronal Weigert-stained section shown in Figures 9-6, 9-7, and 9-8.

Remove one last horizontal slice about 1–2 cm thick through the cerebral hemisphere with the brain knife. This slice should be made through the thalamus just below the anterior tubercle. On the cut surface, review the structures that have been described in this and the preceding chapters. Proceeding from the insular cortex, they are as follows: insular cortex, extreme capsule, claustrum, external capsule, putamen, globus pallidus, anterior limb, genu and posterior limb of the internal capsule, caudate nucleus, lateral ventricle, and thalamus. Refer to the horizontal sections shown in Figures 13-53 and 13-54 to help you identify these structures.

Figure 9-5. Dissection of the medial surface of the right half of the hypothalamus demonstrating the course of the fornix and the mamillothalamic tract.

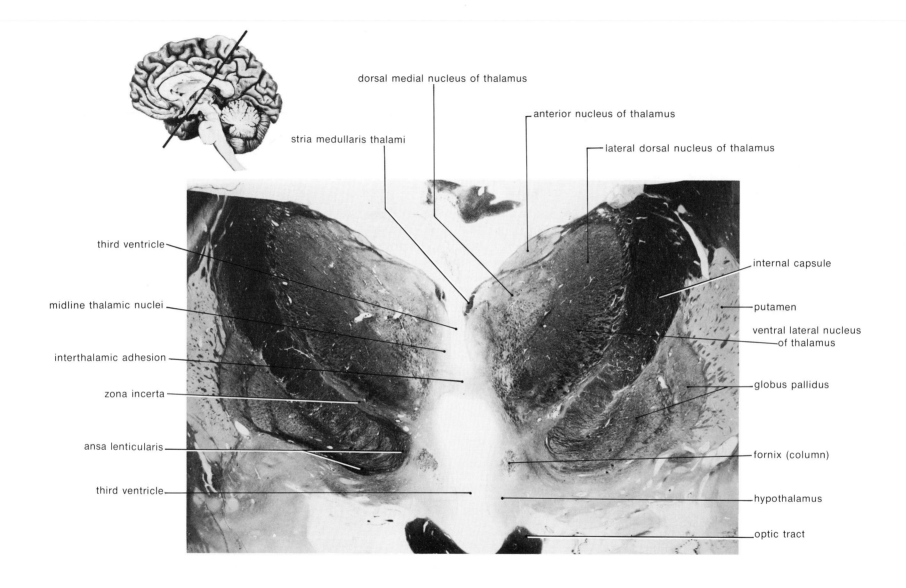

dorsal medial nucleus of thalamus

anterior nucleus of thalamus

lateral dorsal nucleus of thalamus

stria medullaris thalami

third ventricle

internal capsule

midline thalamic nuclei

putamen

ventral lateral nucleus of thalamus

interthalamic adhesion

zona incerta

globus pallidus

ansa lenticularis

fornix (column)

third ventricle

hypothalamus

optic tract

Figure 9-6. Weigert-stained coronal section of the diencephalon and lenticular nuclei taken at the level of the interthalamic adhesion. Subthalamic structures are located ventral to the thalamus and medial to the internal capsule. The solid black line in the key photograph shows the precise plane at which the section was taken.

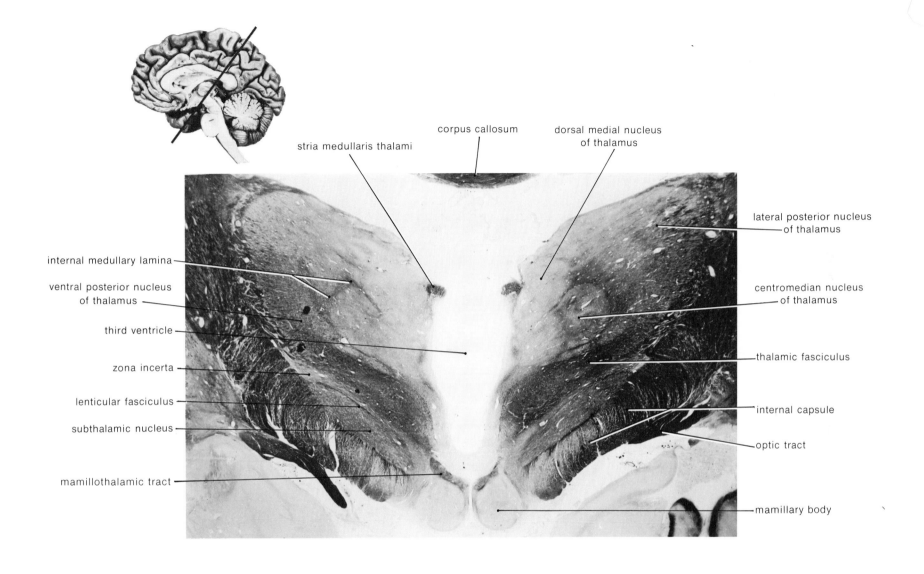

stria medullaris thalami

corpus callosum

dorsal medial nucleus
of thalamus

lateral posterior nucleus
of thalamus

internal medullary lamina

ventral posterior nucleus
of thalamus

third ventricle

zona incerta

lenticular fasciculus

subthalamic nucleus

mamillothalamic tract

centromedian nucleus
of thalamus

thalamic fasciculus

internal capsule

optic tract

mamillary body

Figure 9-7. Weigert-stained section of the diencephalon taken at the level of mamillary bodies of the hypothalamus. Subthalamic structures are located ventral to the
thalamus and medial to the internal capsule. The solid black line in the key photograph shows the precise plane at which the section was taken.

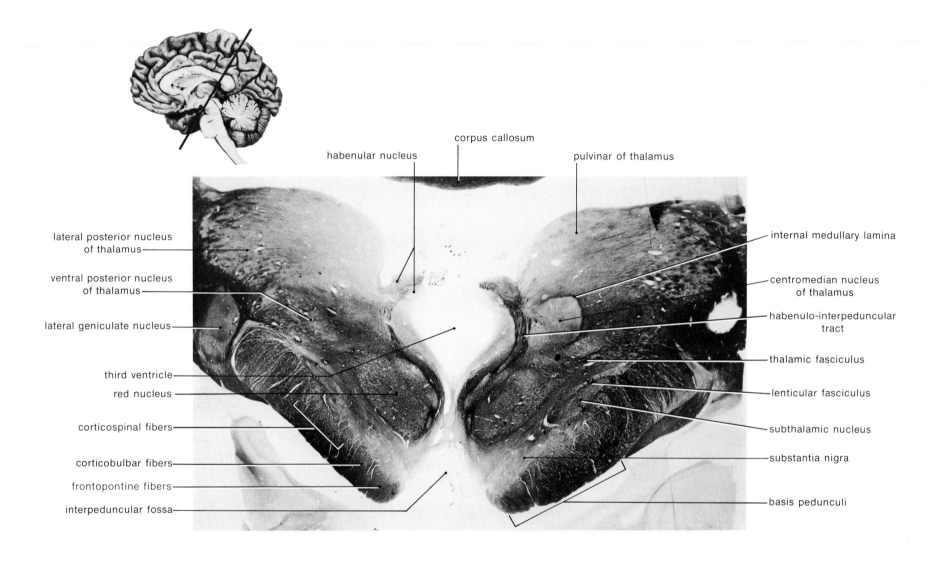

corpus callosum

habenular nucleus

pulvinar of thalamus

lateral posterior nucleus of thalamus

internal medullary lamina

ventral posterior nucleus of thalamus

centromedian nucleus of thalamus

lateral geniculate nucleus

habenulo-interpeduncular tract

third ventricle

thalamic fasciculus

red nucleus

lenticular fasciculus

corticospinal fibers

subthalamic nucleus

corticobulbar fibers

substantia nigra

frontopontine fibers

interpeduncular fossa

basis pedunculi

Figure 9-8. Weigert-stained section taken through the caudal thalamus at the junction between the diencephalon and the midbrain. Structures that comprise the subthalamus are still found in this level. The solid black line in the key photograph shows the precise plane at which the section was taken.

10

Brain Stem and Cranial Nerves

The *brain stem* consists of the midbrain, the pons, and the medulla oblongata. Some authors include the diencephalon as a component of the brain stem. In this text, however, the diencephalon is considered along with the cerebral hemispheres to form the *cerebrum* of the brain. The many and varied structures of the cerebrum are, in some ways, easy to identify because they are often large and well delimited. The brain stem, however, is a comparatively small part of the brain. Its gross features are therefore diminutive and its surface morphology more subtle. It will require careful examination in order to identify the various features described below.

The brain stem may be considered a rostral continuation of the spinal cord. Although surperficially it bears little resemblance to the cord, the internal structure of the two is similar in some respects. As with the spinal cord, the brain stem contains many ascending and descending fiber tracts. It also contains columns of neurons having sensory and motor functions. The sensory columns are located lateral to, and the motor columns medial to, the sulcus limitans. It may be worth noting that in general the sensory nuclei of the brain stem form continuous columns of cells, whereas the motor nuclei are often in discontinuous groups.

Another similarity with the spinal cord is the emergence of 10 pairs of nerves (Fig. 10-1) from the brain stem. These are the *cranial nerves*, of which there are 12 pairs in all. The first two cranial nerves, the olfactory and the optic nerves, have been described in previous chapters dealing with the structure of the cerebrum. The cranial nerves, like the spinal nerves, are classified on the basis of whether their component fibers are afferent (sensory) or efferent (motor), or mixed as well as on the basis of whether the structures innervated are visceral or somatic.

Midbrain

The midbrain is the most rostral division of the brain stem. It is situated between the diencephalon in front and the pons behind. It is derived from the mesencephalon of the embryonic brain, a name that is often used in referring to the midbrain of the adult as well. It is the shortest component of the brain stem (1.5–2.0 cm in length) and similar to the pons and the medulla contains many nuclei as well as ascending and descending fiber tracts. The midbrain consists of dorsal and ventral portions, the *tectum* and the *cerebral peduncles*, respectively, which are organized into symmetric right and left halves. The *cerebral aqueduct* (of Sylvius) traversing the midbrain joins the third ventricle of the diencephalon with the fourth ventricle of the pons and medulla (Fig. 13-1).

The brain stem with attached cerebellum was severed from the cerebrum in Chapter 6. Now view the superior surface of the specimen of the brain stem and cerebellum. This view should be identical to that shown in Figure 11-1. Some of the superior surface of the midbrain is hidden by the overlying anterior lobe of the cerebellum. Retract the anterior lobe of the cerebellum causing it as little damage as possible for it will be examined in the next chapter. This allows you to view the dorsal (posterior) surface of the midbrain. It is com-

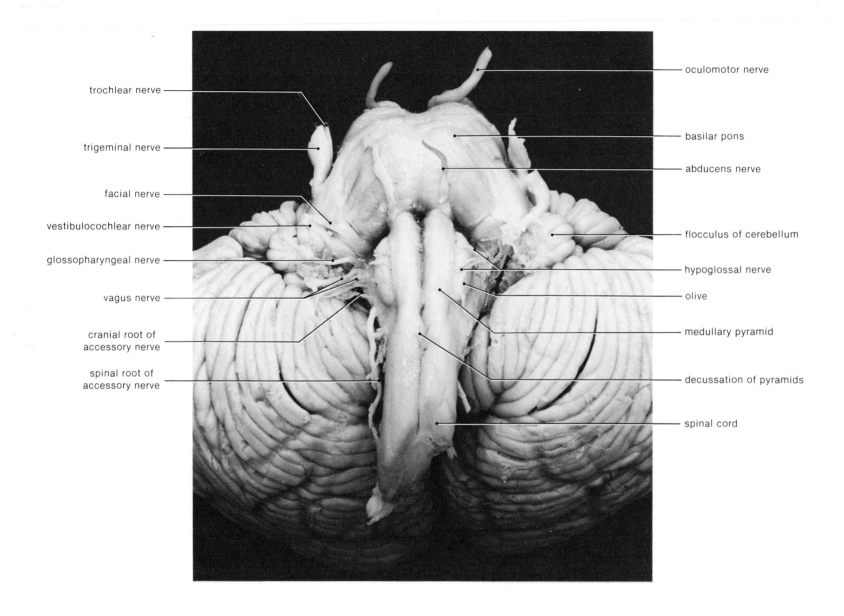

trochlear nerve

trigeminal nerve

facial nerve

vestibulocochlear nerve

glossopharyngeal nerve

vagus nerve

cranial root of
accessory nerve

spinal root of
accessory nerve

oculomotor nerve

basilar pons

abducens nerve

flocculus of cerebellum

hypoglossal nerve

olive

medullary pyramid

decussation of pyramids

spinal cord

posed of two pairs of small eminences, each about 7 mm in diameter, which are known collectively as the *corpora quadrigemina*, or midbrain colliculi. The rostral pair are the *superior colliculi*. They are slightly larger than the more caudal pair, the *inferior colliculi* (see Figs. 11-4 and 13-55). The superior colliculi are formed by the underlying nuclei, which are centers primarily for visual reflexes. These nuclei receive most of their afferents from the visual cortex of the occipital lobe. These afferents reach the superior colliculus by way of a small band of neural tissue called the *brachium of the superior colliculus* (Fig. 10-2). A few fibers from the optic tracts are carried in the superior brachium to terminate also within the superior colliculus. In addition to these, the spinotectal tract carrying information from cutaneous receptors in the body also terminates in the superior colliculus. When the brain stem was separated from the cerebrum in Chapter 6 the superior brachium was cut, for it is located at the junction of the diencephalon with the midbrain. However, you may be able to identify a remnant of the superior brachium attached to the lateral geniculate body on the inferior surface of the pulvinar of the thalamus. In its course toward the superior colliculus it partly overlaps the medial geniculate body.

The inferior colliculi are composed of neurons that are associated with the auditory pathway (Fig. 10-4; see also Figs. 11-4 and 13-39). Each also possesses a brachium, the *brachium of the inferior colliculus*, which runs ventral and lateral to the superior colliculus to terminate in the medial geniculate body of the thalamus. It conveys fibers from the lateral lemniscus and inferior colliculus to the medial geniculate nucleus.

You will recall that the medial geniculate nucleus, also located on the under surface of the pulvinar, is a relay nucleus in the auditory pathway. Identify a slight triangular swelling on the dorsolateral surface of the midbrain just caudal to the inferior colliculus. This is the *lemniscal trigone*, which overlaps the superior cerebellar peduncle in an oblique fashion. This swelling is produced by the underlying *lateral lemniscus*, which is the main auditory pathway within the brain stem; its constituent fibers synapse with neurons of the inferior colliculus and medial geniculate nucleus. The superior and inferior colliculi and their brachia constitute what is known as the *tectum* or the roof plate of the midbrain.

Immediately behind the inferior colliculus identify the slender *trochlear nerve* (CN IV) emerging from the midbrain lateral to the superior medullary velum. It is the only cranial nerve that emerges from the dorsal surface of the brain stem (see Fig. 11-4). This nerve arises from the *trochlear nucleus*, which is located ventral to the cerebral aqueduct in the periaqueductal gray matter at the level of the inferior colliculus (Fig. 10-4). The axons from this nucleus curve around the central or periaqueductal gray of the caudal midbrain toward the dorsal surface, where they decussate in the superior medullary velum. After leaving the brain stem, the nerve encircles the cerebral peduncle to assume a ventral position similar to that of the other cranial nerves. The trochlear nerve is a purely somatic efferent nerve innervating one of the extraocular muscles, the *superior oblique muscle*.

Those portions of the midbrain exclusive of the tectum are the *cerebral peduncles*. Now examine the cut surface of the midbrain made earlier at its junction with the diencephalon (Fig. 10-2; see also Figs. 11-1 and 13-56). Each cerebral peduncle is composed of a ventral portion, the *basis pedunculi* (often called the *crus cerebri*), and a more dorsal part, the *tegmentum*. The tegmentum is separated from the basis pedunculi by a crescent-shaped pigmented nucleus, the *substantia nigra*, so named because many of the neurons of this nucleus contain a dark melanin pigment. On this same cut surface identify within the tegmentum an oval region about 5 mm in diameter just dorsal and medial to the substantia nigra, which is only slightly darker than the surrounding tissue. This is the cut surface of the *red nucleus*. This nucleus and the substantia nigra are important motor nuclei.

The massive right and left basis pedunculi are easily seen on the ventral (anterior) surface of the midbrain. Emerging from each cerebral hemisphere, they converge as they descend toward the pons. Their surface is corrugated in the longitudinal direction. They contain projection fibers that descend from extensive areas of the cerebral cortex. These fibers, which form the corona radiata, traverse the internal capsule and become concentrated in the basis pedunculi (Figs. 10-2, 10-3, 10-4, and 10-12). They project to the motor nuclei of some of the cranial nerves, the brain stem reticular formation, the nuclei pontis, and the spinal cord. The two crura are separated by a deep midline depression, the *interpeduncular fossa* (Figs. 8-4, 10-2, 10-

---

Figure 10-1.   Ventral view of the brain stem with attached cerebellum showing the location of the entry or emergence of 10 of the 12 pairs of cranial nerves.

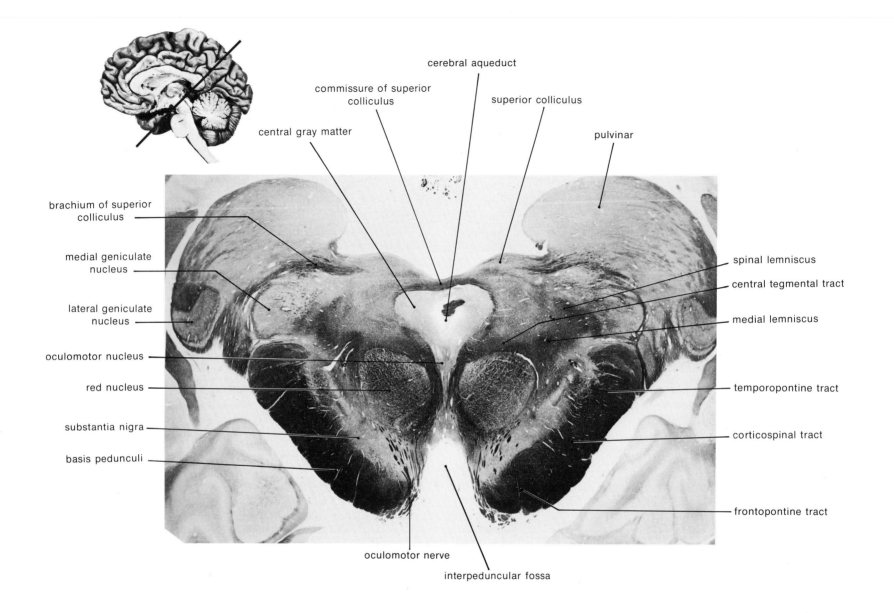

cerebral aqueduct

commissure of superior
colliculus

superior colliculus

central gray matter

pulvinar

brachium of superior
colliculus

medial geniculate
nucleus

lateral geniculate
nucleus

oculomotor nucleus

red nucleus

substantia nigra

basis pedunculi

spinal lemniscus

central tegmental tract

medial lemniscus

temporopontine tract

corticospinal tract

frontopontine tract

oculomotor nerve

interpeduncular fossa

82

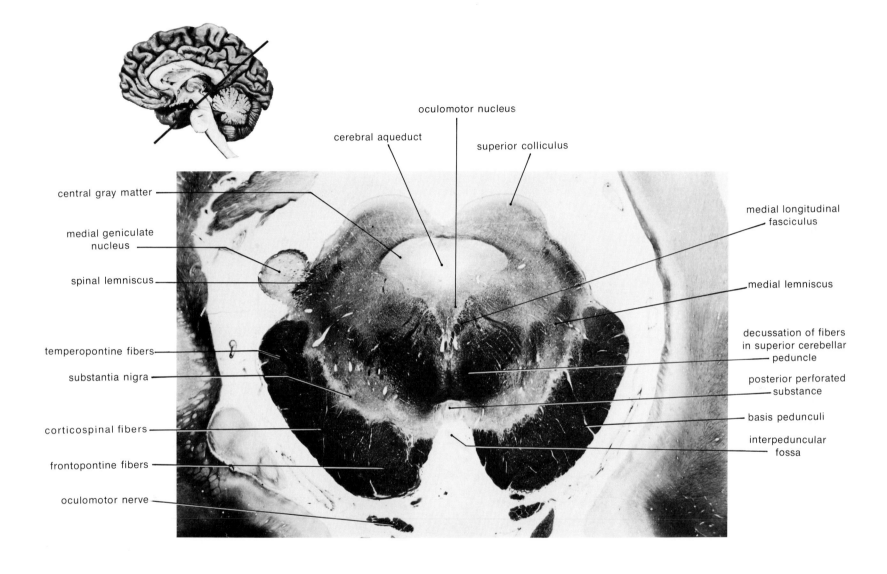

oculomotor nucleus

cerebral aqueduct

superior colliculus

central gray matter

medial longitudinal fasciculus

medial geniculate nucleus

spinal lemniscus

medial lemniscus

temperopontine fibers

decussation of fibers in superior cerebellar peduncle

substantia nigra

posterior perforated substance

corticospinal fibers

basis pedunculi

interpeduncular fossa

frontopontine fibers

oculomotor nerve

Figure 10-2. Weigert-stained transverse section of the brain stem taken at the junction of the midbrain with the diencephalon. The solid black line in the key photograph shows the precise plane at which the section was taken.

Figure 10-3. Weigert-stained transverse section through the midbrain at the level of the superior colliculus. The solid black line in the key photograph shows the precise plane at which the section was taken.

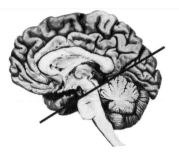

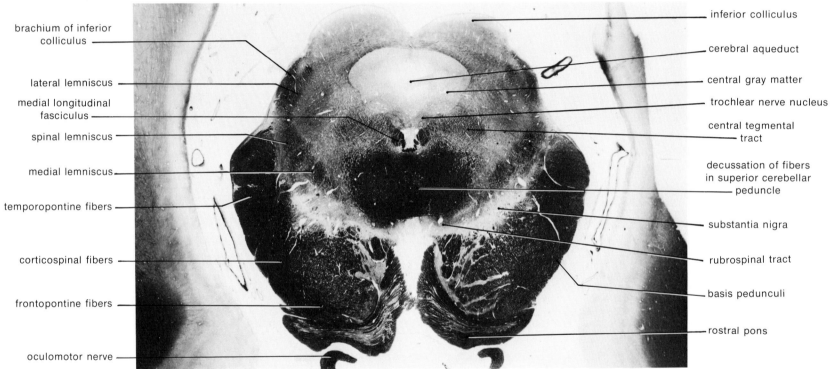

brachium of inferior colliculus

lateral lemniscus

medial longitudinal fasciculus

spinal lemniscus

medial lemniscus

temporopontine fibers

corticospinal fibers

frontopontine fibers

oculomotor nerve

inferior colliculus

cerebral aqueduct

central gray matter

trochlear nerve nucleus

central tegmental tract

decussation of fibers in superior cerebellar peduncle

substantia nigra

rubrospinal tract

basis pedunculi

rostral pons

3, and 10-12). The surface of this fossa has a punctate appearance similar to that of the anterior perforated substance. It is called the *posterior perforated substance* because it is penetrated by central branches of the posterior cerebral artery supplying the deep structures of the tegmentum, the subthalamic and mamillary regions, and the medial part of the basis pedunculi.

The *oculomotor nerve* (CN III) emerges from the interpeduncular fossa of the midbrain along the medial surface of each crus cerebri. It passes between the superior cerebellar and posterior cerebral arteries and then curves laterally and forward toward the orbit. The oculomotor is the largest of the nerves supplying the extrinsic muscles of the eye. Its axons arise from the *oculomotor nuclear complex* located just ventral to the aqueduct at the level of the superior colliculus (Figs. 10-2 and 10-3). This is a complex of cell groups that provide motor fibers to the levator palpebrae superioris muscle and to all of the extraocular muscles (superior rectus, inferior rectus, medial rectus, and inferior oblique) except the lateral rectus and the superior oblique muscles. In addition, the oculomotor nuclear complex includes the accessory oculomotor nucleus, a small nucleus that contributes parasympathetic preganglionic fibers to the ciliary ganglion via the oculomotor nerve. The postganglionic fibers are distributed to the intrinsic muscles of the eye, the ciliary muscle and the sphincter pupillae. This component of the accessory oculomotor nucleus that gives origin to the preganglionic parasympathetics bears the eponym of the *Edinger–Westphal nucleus* after the names of two prominent German neurologists.

Pons

The pons is the stout bridge of gray and white matter about 2.5 cm long that lies between the midbrain and the medulla. It is composed of two distinct regions. The dorsal portion is similar in some respects to the midbrain and medulla in that it contains certain nuclear masses and shares certain fiber tracts with the rest of the brain stem. The dorsal portion of the pons is called the *pontine tegmentum*, and its

Figure 10-4. Weigert-stained transverse section through the midbrain at the level of the inferior colliculus. The solid black line in the key photograph shows the precise plane at which the section was taken.

surface is seen only as the floor of the fourth ventricle, which will be examined in the next chapter. The cerebellum is located above the pons and perched on the three cerebellar peduncles. It conceals the dorsal surface of the pons. The ventral part of the pons is called the *basilar portion of the pons.* The greatest development of this region occurs in mammals and is concomitant with the development of the cerebral hemispheres and the neocerebellum; it is especially prominent in the human brain. It functions primarily as a cell station in the massive projection system from the cerebral cortex of one side to the cerebellar cortex of the contralateral side. Transversely oriented pontocerebellar fibers make up the entire middle cerebellar peduncles. These fibers, along with the nuclei pontis and the longitudinally oriented conticopontine and corticospinal motor fibers, constitute the basilar portion of the pons (Figs. 10-5 and 10-6). The ventral surface of the pons is corrugated in a transverse direction, and there is a shallow longitudinal sulcus, the *basilar sulcus* in the midline. This sulcus lodges the basilar artery. The caudal limit of the basilar pons is marked by a prominent transverse sulcus, the *bulbopontine sulcus* (Fig. 10-1).

The pontine tegmentum contains in whole or in part the nuclei of four of the cranial nerves (CN, V, VI, VII, and VIII). The largest cranial nerve, the *trigeminal nerve* (CN V), emerges from the ventrolateral surface of the pons at its junction with the middle cerebellar peduncle (Fig. 10-1). It consists of a small motor root and a large sensory root. Fibers of the sensory root are the central processes of cells within the *trigeminal* (semilunar) *ganglion.* Their peripheral processes enter the *ophthalmic, maxillary,* and *mandibular* divisions of the trigeminal nerve. The trigeminal nerve is the sensory nerve of the face, most of the scalp, the nasal and oral cavities, the teeth, the frontal and maxillary sinuses, the dura mater of the middle and anterior cranial fossae, the anterior wall of the external acoustic meatus, and part of a tympanic membrane. The mandibular division also conveys fibers of a proprioceptive nature from structures that include the temporomandibular joint and the muscles of mastication (masseter, temporalis, and pterygoid muscles). The central processes of these sensory neurons terminate in one or more of the three sensory nuclei that form the *central trigeminal nuclei.* These nuclei form a continuous column of cells in the dorsolateral part of the brain stem extending from the level of the superior colliculus to the second cervical segment of the spinal cord. The *pontine* or *principal sen-*

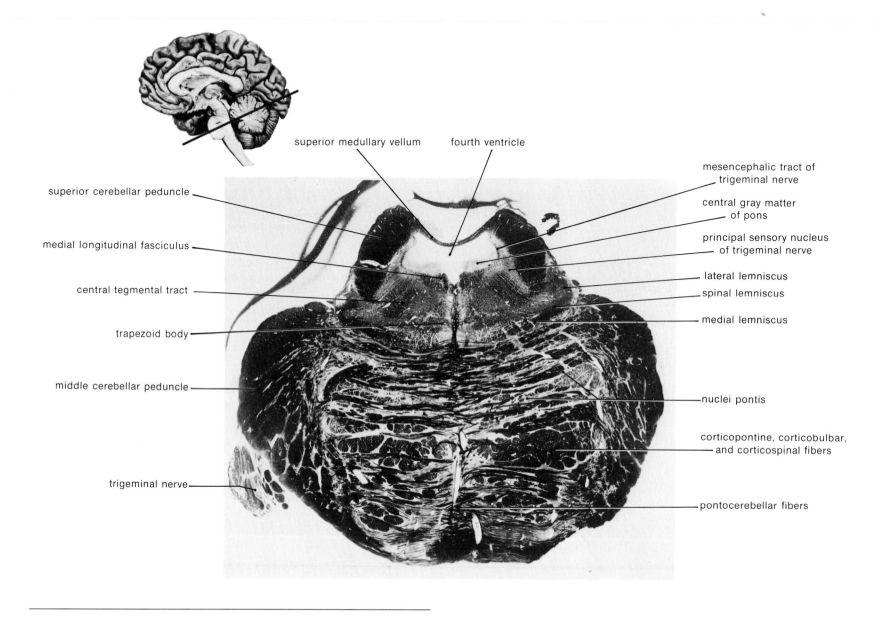

superior medullary vellum   fourth ventricle

mesencephalic tract of trigeminal nerve

superior cerebellar peduncle

central gray matter of pons

medial longitudinal fasciculus

principal sensory nucleus of trigeminal nerve

central tegmental tract

lateral lemniscus

spinal lemniscus

medial lemniscus

trapezoid body

middle cerebellar peduncle

nuclei pontis

corticopontine, corticobulbar, and corticospinal fibers

trigeminal nerve

pontocerebellar fibers

Figure 10-5. Weigert-stained transverse section through the rostral portion of the pons. The solid black line in the key photograph shows the precise plane at which the section was taken.

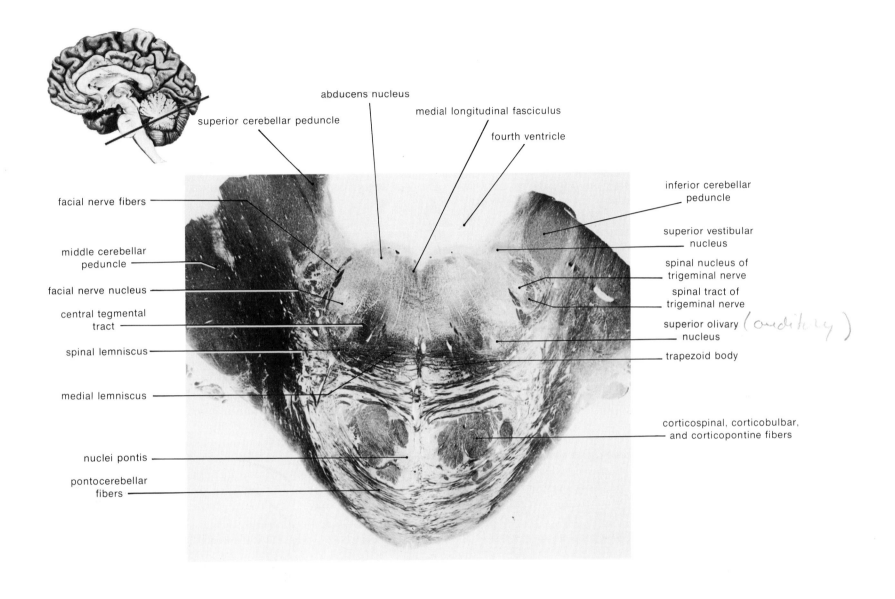

superior cerebellar peduncle

abducens nucleus

medial longitudinal fasciculus

fourth ventricle

inferior cerebellar peduncle

facial nerve fibers

superior vestibular nucleus

middle cerebellar peduncle

spinal nucleus of trigeminal nerve

facial nerve nucleus

spinal tract of trigeminal nerve

central tegmental tract

superior olivary (auditory) nucleus

spinal lemniscus

trapezoid body

medial lemniscus

corticospinal, corticobulbar, and corticopontine fibers

nuclei pontis

pontocerebellar fibers

Figure 10-6. Weigert-stained transverse section through the caudal portion of the pons. The solid black line in the key photograph shows the precise plane at which the section was taken.

87

sory nucleus lies in the dorsolateral part of the pontine tegmentum deep to the superior and middle cerebellar peduncles; it is mainly associated with tactile sensation. The slender *mesencephalic* nucleus extends rostrally from the principal sensory nucleus to the level of the superior colliculus in the lateral periaqueductal gray of the midbrain (Fig. 10-5); it is associated with proprioceptive sensations from the muscles of mastication. The *spinal nucleus* of the *trigeminal nerve* extends from the pontine nucleus to the upper cervical segments of the spinal cord, where it becomes continuous with the *substantia gelatinosa*. It is concerned primarily with pain and thermal sensation as well as tactile sensibility. On their descent through the pons and the medulla, sensory root fibers destined to terminate in the spinal nucleus form a band called the *spinal tract of the trigeminal nerve,* which overlies the nucleus dorsolaterally (Figs. 10-6 to 10-12; 13-44, and 13-60). From the three sensory nuclei, most secondary trigeminal fibers project to the ventral posterior medial nucleus of the thalamus, from which fibers are then relayed via the thalamic radiations to the primary somesthetic cortex of the post central gyrus. Fibers from the mesencephalic nucleus project to the motor nucleus of the trigeminal nerve and cerebellum as well.

The *motor nucleus of the trigeminal nerve* is located medial to the principal sensory nucleus in the dorsolateral pontine tegmentum. It provides motor innervation to the muscles of mastication and to the tensor tympani and tensor veli palatini muscles via the mandibular branch of the trigeminal nerve.

A certain type of pathology involving the sensory trigeminal nerve called *trigeminal neuralgia,* or *tic douloureux,* is sufficiently common to warrant brief mention at this time. It constitutes a severe type of stabbing pain along one or more of the three peripheral divisions of the nerve. The pain may last a few seconds in each paroxysm and may be induced by tapping the skin of the face. In spite of the fact that the precise etiology of this excruciating pain is still uncertain, a vareity of medical and neurosurgical procedures have been employed in the treatment of such patients.

The nucleus of the *abducens nerve* (CN VI) is located beneath the floor of the fourth ventricle in the medial portion of the pons. It underlies the median eminence between the sulcus limitans and the median sulcus. The efferent fibers of the facial nerve loop around it as the *internal genu of the facial nerve* (Fig. 10-6). The axons arising from the abducens nucleus course ventrally through the pons and emerge on the ventral surface of the brain stem from the bulbopontine sulcus between the pons and the medullary pyramid (Fig. 10-1). The abducens nerve ultimately enters the orbit and supplies the lateral rectus muscle of the eye.

The central nuclei of the *facial nerve* (CN VII) consist of two motor nuclei and one sensory nucleus located in the posterior part of the pontine tegmentum and medulla oblongata, respectively (Fig. 10-6). It can be said that there are two sensory nuclei if one considers the fact that some sensory fibers conveyed in the nerve terminate in the spinal nucleus of the trigeminal nerve. The fibers of the sensory root of the facial nerve, which is given a separate name, the *nervus intermedius,* arise from the cells of the *geniculate ganglion.* Their central processes enter the brain stem at the *pontomedullocerebellar angle* just lateral to the abducens nerve (Fig. 10-1). These fibers traverse the basilar pons and terminate in the spinal nucleus of the trigeminal nerve as well as in the rostral end of the soilitary nucleus. The latter nucleus is a column of cells that begins at the lower border of the pons and continues caudally through the medulla (Figs. 10-7 to 10-9). Those fibers of the intermediate nerve that end in the spinal nucleus of the trigeminal nerve convey cutaneous sensation from the skin of the auricle, from a small area of skin behind the ear, and from the external auditory meatus and part of the tympanic membrane. Those fibers terminating in the *solitary nucleus* transmit impulses related to taste sensation from the anterior two-thirds of the tongue.

The fibers of the motor root of the facial nerve arise from the large *motor nucleus,* which lies ventral and medial to the spinal nucleus of the trigeminal nerve in the caudal part of the pontine tegmentum (Fig. 10-6). The axons of the neurons in the motor nucleus pass dorsally toward the floors of the fourth ventricle medial to the abducens nucleus. They curve laterally over the anterior end of the abducens nucleus and come to lie between it and the floor of the ventricle, thus forming the genu of the facial nerve. The fibers then pass ventrally and laterally through the pons to emerge from the brain stem along with the sensory root (Fig. 10-1). The motor root

Figure 10-7. Weigart-stained transverse section through the rostral portion of the medulla oblongata. The solid black line in the key photograph shows the precise plane at which the section was taken.

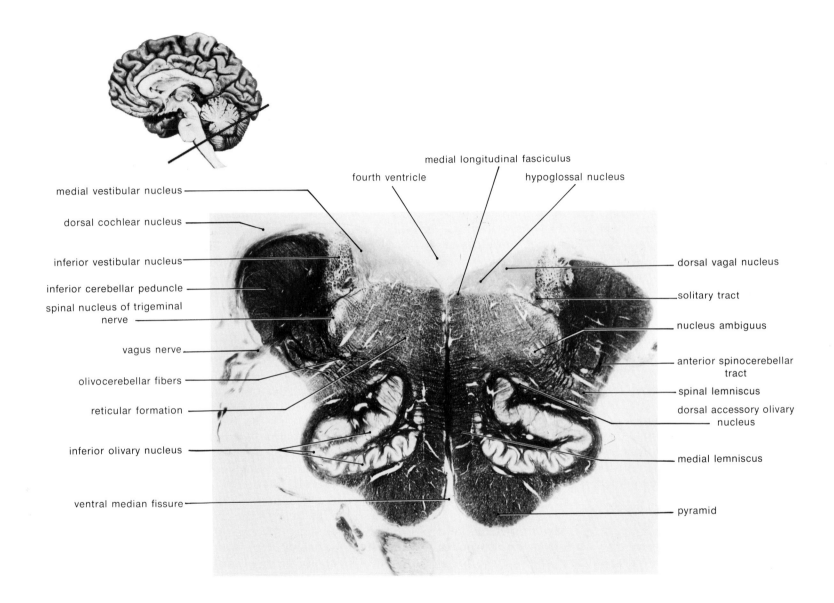

medial longitudinal fasciculus

fourth ventricle   hypoglossal nucleus

medial vestibular nucleus

dorsal cochlear nucleus

inferior vestibular nucleus

inferior cerebellar peduncle

spinal nucleus of trigeminal nerve

vagus nerve

olivocerebellar fibers

reticular formation

inferior olivary nucleus

ventral median fissure

dorsal vagal nucleus

solitary tract

nucleus ambiguus

anterior spinocerebellar tract

spinal lemniscus

dorsal accessory olivary nucleus

medial lemniscus

pyramid

innervates the muscles of facial expression, the muscles of the scalp and auricle, the buccinator and platysma muscles, the posterior belly of the digastric, and the stylohyoid and stapedius muscles. The facial nerve also contains efferent parasympathetic fibers that arise from the *superior salivatory* and *lacrimal nuclei* located close to the caudal end of the facial motor nucleus at the pontomedullary junction. These preganglionic fibers are conveyed in the nervus intermedius to the submandibular and pterygopalatine ganglia. The postganglionic fibers innervate the submandibular and sublingual salivary glands and the lacrimal, nasal, and palatine glands, respectively. For this reason, the nervus intermedius cannot be called a solely sensory nerve.

Lesions of the central or peripheral divisions of the facial nerve result in varying constellations of sensory and motor deficits depending upon the location and extent of the lesion. The more obvious symptoms are loss of taste sensation from the anterior two-thirds of the tongue and paresis or paralysis of the muscles of facial expression (Bell's palsy).

The *vestibulocochlear nerve* (CN VIII) emerges from the brain stem in the bulbopontine sulcus just lateral to the facial nerve. It is, in fact, composed of two nerves, the *vestibular* and the *cochlear* nerves. The vestibular nerve is formed from the central processes of the neurons in the *vestibular ganglion* (of Scarpa). The peripheral processes of these neurons end around the sensory hair cells of the maculae of the saccule and utricle and the cristae of the semicircular ducts. The central processes branch soon after they enter the brain stem and terminate in the complex of vestibular nuclei underlying the vestibular area in the floor of the most lateral part of the fourth ventricle in the pons and the medulla (Figs. 10-6 to 10-8). Some of these afferent fibers continue uninterrupted into the cerebellum via the inferior cerebellar peduncle.

There are four vestibular nuclei *superior, inferior, medial,* and *lateral* (of Deiters) (Figs. 10-6 to 10-8). From these nuclei a variety of pathways arise. The *lateral vestibulospinal tract* arises from the neurons of the ispilateral lateral nucleus and descends the length of the spinal cord, terminating on interneurons or motor neurons of the anterior horn to maintain the tonus of the axial and appendicular musculature for posture and balance in response to vestibular stimulation. The *medial vestibulospinal tract* arises primarily from the medial vestibular nucleus. It descends in the spinal cord both ipsilaterally and contralaterally to cervical levels only as a component of the descending *medial longitudinal fasciculus.* It performs the same function with respect to the muscles of the neck as does the lateral vestibulospinal tract for the trunk and the upper and lower limbs. The medial longitudinal fasciculus is both a crossed and uncrossed composite bundle of fibers, which at brain stem levels is located near the midline below the cerebral aqueduct and the fourth ventricle (Figs. 10-3 to 10-9). It is composed of ascending and descending fibers. Ascending fibers arise from neruons in all four vestibular nuclei and project mainly to the motor nuclei innervating the extraocular muscles, thus providing for movements of the eyes in response to vestibular stimulation.

Vestibular stimulation is perceived consciously, but the precise location of a primary vestibular area within the cerebral cortex is still a matter of controversy. It has been suggested that such an area is located in the superior temporal gyrus caudal to the auditory area. Another vestibular area has been located near the head area of the postcentral gyrus.

One of the signs of disease of the vestibular system is *nystagmus,* which is a rhythmic conjugate movement of the eyes characterized by a slow movement in one direction and a fast movement in the opposite direction. Although nystagmus can be induced in normal individuals by a variety of means, its spontaneous appearance is usually pathological.

The *cochlear nerve* is composed of the central processes of the neurons in the *cochlear* (spiral) *ganglion* in the bony spiral lamina of the cochlea. The peripheral processes of these ganglion cells terminate around the base of the sensory hair cells of the organ of Corti. Upon entering the brain stem, the centrally directed processes bifurcate, sending one branch to the *dorsal cochlear nucleus* and one to the *ventral cochlear nucleus.* These nuclei are located at the junction of the pons with the medulla on the root of the inferior cerebellar peduncle (Fig. 10-7). They give rise to the ascending auditory pathway. Although this pathway is predominantly contralateral, there is a significant ipsilateral component. The pathway is characterized by synapses in several brain stem nuclei: the superior olivary nucleus, the

Figure 10-8. Weigert-stained transverse section through the open portion of the medulla oblongata at the midolivary level. The solid black line in the key photograph shows the precise plane at which the section was taken.

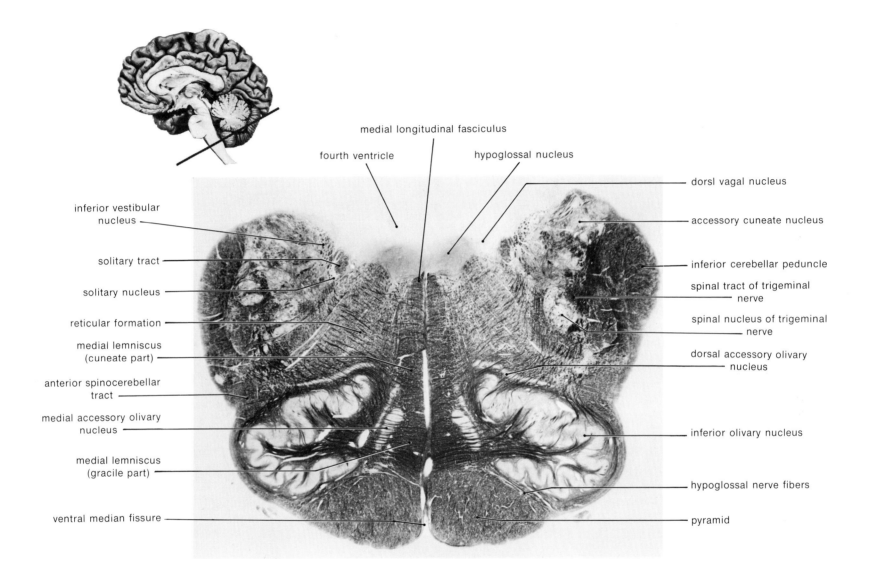

medial longitudinal fasciculus

fourth ventricle

hypoglossal nucleus

dorsl vagal nucleus

accessory cuneate nucleus

inferior vestibular nucleus

inferior cerebellar peduncle

solitary tract

spinal tract of trigeminal nerve

solitary nucleus

spinal nucleus of trigeminal nerve

reticular formation

medial lemniscus (cuneate part)

dorsal accessory olivary nucleus

anterior spinocerebellar tract

medial accessory olivary nucleus

inferior olivary nucleus

medial lemniscus (gracile part)

hypoglossal nerve fibers

ventral median fissure

pyramid

nucleus of the lateral lemniscus, the inferior colliculus, and the medial geniculate nucleus. It ultimately projects from the medial geniculate nucleus via the auditory radiations of the internal capsule to the auditory cortex (Heschl's convolutions) of the temporal lobe. In the brain stem, the auditory pathway is called the *lateral lemniscus*. By the time it reaches the midbrain, the lateral lemniscus is located superficially beneath the lemniscal trigone just caudal to the inferior colliculus.

Apart from this pathway, some fibers of the cochlear nuclei project to the reticular formation and to the motor nuclei of cranial nerves III, IV, V, VI, and VII, mediating reflexes in response to auditory stimuli. Lesions located in the cochlear ganglion or the cochlear nerve before it enters the brain stem will result in deafness in the corresponding ear. However, because of the significant bilaterality of the central auditory pathway, from there onward, lesions involving the lateral lemniscus, inferior colliculus, medial geniculate nucleus, or auditory cortex on one side result only in a diminution of hearing in the contralateral ear.

The cochlear nerve also contains efferent fibers that form the *olivocochlear tract* and that arise from the superior olivary nucleus and terminate in the organ of Corti.

Medulla

The medulla is the rostral continuation of the spinal cord. There is no abrupt line of demarcation between the two; the junction is arbitrarily considered to be along a transverse plane corresponding approximately with the level of the foramen magnum. The medulla extends forward from here for a distance of about 3 cm to the caudal border of the pons, increasing in its transverse diameter as it ascends (Fig. 10-1).

The medulla is divided into symmetric right and left halves by the *ventral median fissure* (Fig. 10-1) and the *dorsal median sulcus* (Fig. 11-4). These grooves are extensions of those on the ventral (anterior) and the dorsal (posterior) surfaces of the spinal cord. The elongated eminence immediately lateral to the ventral median fissure is the *medullary pyramid*. It marks the position of the underlying corticospinal tract, which, together with the *corticobulbar tract* ending on brain stem nuclei, constitutes the *pyramidal motor pathway*. The ventral median fissure is interrupted about 2.5–3 cm caudal to the bulbopontine sulcus by stout bundles of fibers crossing diagonally from one side to the other (Fig. 10-1). This is the *decussation* of the *pyramids*, where most (70–90%) of the corticospinal fibers of the pyramid cross the midline to enter the contralateral lateral funiculus of the spinal cord. In some brain specimens the pyramidal decussation may not be present, the medulla having been transected rostral to it when the brain was removed from the skull at autopsy. If the medulla in your specimen is complete, you may locate the pyramidal decussation by inserting a blunt probe into the ventral median fissure and running the tip of the probe caudally until its further passage is obstructed. Gentle separation of the pyramids at this level will reveal the decussating bundles.

Just lateral to the pyramid identify a shallow longitudinal depression, the *ventrolateral sulcus*. In this sulcus notice the many small rootlets of the *hypoglossal nerve* (CN XII) that emerge in a line between the pyramid and the olive. The *olive* is a prominent oval swelling about 12 mm in length on the ventrolateral surface of the medulla (Figs. 10-1 and 10-12). This swelling is caused by the underlying *inferior olivary nucleus*, which in cross section has an undulating folded appearance of an old cloth purse (Figs. 11-7, 11-8, and 11-9). This nucleus receives afferents from muscle and joint receptors, and from the red nucleus and the sensorimotor cortex. It projects to the cerebellar cortex via the inferior cerebellar peduncle.

The dorsal curved edge of the olive is marked by a shallow depression, the *retroolivary sulcus*. It is along this sulcus and in the narrow area between it and the inferior cerebellar peduncle that the rootlets of cranial nerves IX, X, and XI emerge from the medulla.

The first four or five of these small rootlets belong to the *glossopharyngeal nerve* (CN IX) (Fig. 10-1). This cranial nerve subserves a variety of sensory and motor functions related to the head area. It provides the sensory innervation to the taste buds of the posterior one-third of the tongue. The central processes from the *inferior* (petrosal) *ganglion* of cranial nerve IX enter the medulla to form part of the *solitary tract* and terminate in the adjacent *solitary nucleus* (Figs. 10-7, 10-8, and 10-9). As stated previously, the taste fibers of the

Figure 10-9. Weigert-stained section through the medulla oblongata at the caudal limit of the fourth ventricle near the obex. The solid black line in the key photograph shows the precise plane at which the section was taken.

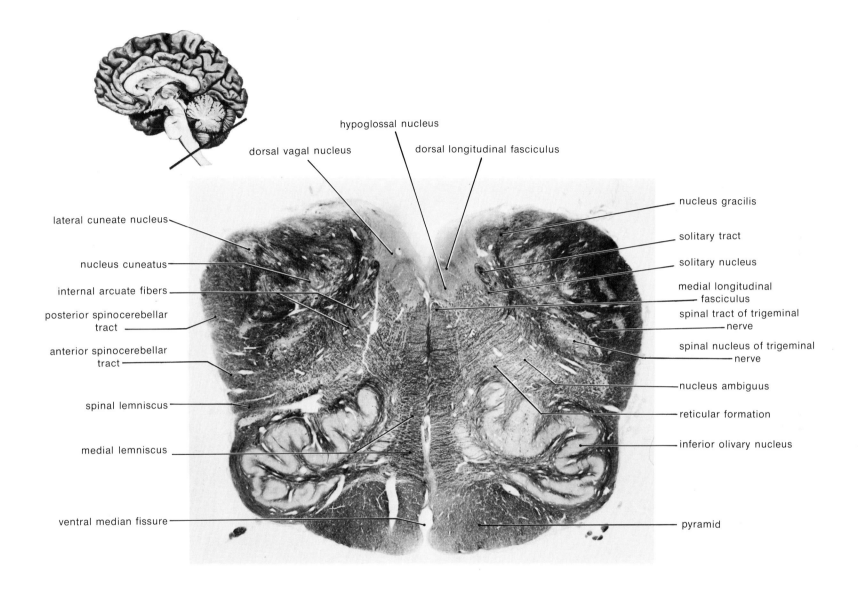

hypoglossal nucleus

dorsal vagal nucleus

dorsal longitudinal fasciculus

nucleus gracilis

lateral cuneate nucleus

solitary tract

nucleus cuneatus

solitary nucleus

internal arcuate fibers

medial longitudinal fasciculus

posterior spinocerebellar tract

spinal tract of trigeminal nerve

anterior spinocerebellar tract

spinal nucleus of trigeminal nerve

nucleus ambiguus

spinal lemniscus

reticular formation

medial lemniscus

inferior olivary nucleus

ventral median fissure

pyramid

facial nerve also terminate here. The rostral portion of the solitary nucleus is therefore often referred to as the *gustatory nucleus.* Cutaneous sensation from the external ear, a small area of skin behind the ear, the acoustic meatus, and the tympanic membrane is also carried in the glossopharyngeal nerve. The central processes of these fibers probably terminate within the spinal nucleus of the trigeminal nerve. The glossopharyngeal nerve also carries the sensations of pain and temperature from the mucous membranes of the posterior part of the tongue, the tonsil, the upper pharynx, and the eustachian tube. It carries impulses from the baroreceptors of the carotid sinus and is therefore involved in the carotid sinus reflex, which functions to lower blood pressure by slowing the heart rate in response to increased carotid arterial pressure.

The preganglionic parasympathetic component of the glossopharyngeal nerve arises from the *inferior salivatory nucleus,* which is a relatively small group of cells near the rostral pole of the *nucleus ambiguus* in the medulla (Fig. 10-7). From these cells arise the preganglionic parasympathetic fibers providing ultimately for the secretomotor innervation of the parotid salivary gland.

The motor component arises from the nucleus ambiguus, which is a column of cells in the medulla dorsal to the inferior olivary nucleus (Figs. 10-7 and 10-9). This is a common efferent nucleus that is shared by the vagus and the accessory nerves. The fibers that arise from the rostral pole of this nucleus leave the medulla in the glossopharyngeal nerve and innervate the stylopharyngeus muscle.

The next six to eight rootlets immediately caudal to the glossopharyngeal belong to the *vagus nerve* (CN X). This nerve has some things in common with the glossopharyngeal nerve: It has the same types of component fibers and it shares some of the sensory and motor nuclei in the medulla with the glossopharyngeal nerve. The vagus nerve provides the sensory innervation to the skin of the external ear, a small area of skin behind the ear, the external acoustic meatus, and the tympanic membrane—the same areas provided by a few fibers of the glossopharyngeal nerve. The central processes of these neurons, similar to those of the glossopharyngeal, terminate within the spinal nucleus to the trigeminal nerve. The general sensory innervation of the esophagus, the pharynx, the larynx, and the thoracic and abdominal viscera is also carried in the vagus nerve. The primary sensory neurons are in the *inferior* (nodose) *ganglion;* the central processes of these neurons may terminate either in the

spinal nucleus of the trigeminal nerve or in the solitary nucleus (Figs. 10-7, 10-8, and 10-9). A few fibers carrying sensation of taste from the epiglottis are also included in the vagus nerve; such fibers form part of the solitary tract and end within the solitary nucleus.

The preganglionic parasympathetic innervation of the glands and muscle of the thoracic and abdominal viscera derives from the *dorsal nucleus of the vagus nerve,* which lies beneath the vagal triangle in the floor of the fourth ventricle (Figs. 10-7, 10-8, 10-9, and 11-4). A second motor nucleus of the vagus, the *nucleus ambiguus,* provides the motor innervation of the striated (branchiomeric) muscles of the larynx, the pharynx, and the upper part of the esophagus. It is therefore essential for the normal gag and swallowing reflexes.

Because the glossopharyngeal and vagus nerves serve many functions, lesions in their central complex of nuclei will result in a variety of symptomatology. Such may occur following occlusion of the posterior inferior cerebellar artery (lateral medullary or Wallenberg's syndrome). Among the symptoms may be loss of taste from the posterior part of the tongue, difficulties in swallowing, paralysis of the vocal cords, and tachycardia, to mention but a few.

The *accessory nerve* (CN XI) consists of a cranial division and a spinal division. The last three or four rootlets emerging from the retroolivary sulcus caudal to the vagus are those of the cranial division of this nerve. They arise from the most caudal portion of the nucleus ambiguus and join the vagus nerve innervating the intrinsic muscles of the larynx and the muscles of the soft palate. The spinal portion of the nerve arises from a column of cells (accessory nucleus) in the anterior horn of the upper five to six cervical segments of the cord (Fig. 10-11). These motor fibers leave the cord in the lateral funiculus midway between the ventral and dorsal roots. They fuse to form the *spinal root of the accessory nerve,* which ascends in the vertebral canal and enters the cranial cavity through the foramen magnum. It joins with the cranial root for a short distance only to leave it again after passing through the jugular foramen. The spinal root fibers continue their descent to innervate the trapezius and sterno-

Figure 10-10. Weigert-stained transverse section through the closed portion of the medulla oblongata at the decussation of the fibers of the medial lemniscus. The solid black line in the key photograph shows the precise plane at which the section was taken.

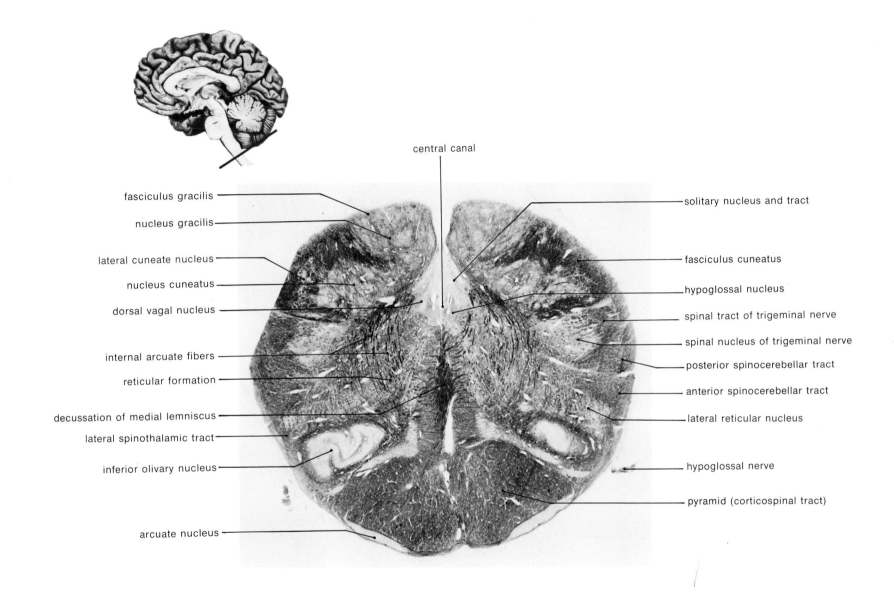

central canal

fasciculus gracilis

nucleus gracilis

lateral cuneate nucleus

nucleus cuneatus

dorsal vagal nucleus

internal arcuate fibers

reticular formation

decussation of medial lemniscus

lateral spinothalamic tract

inferior olivary nucleus

arcuate nucleus

solitary nucleus and tract

fasciculus cuneatus

hypoglossal nucleus

spinal tract of trigeminal nerve

spinal nucleus of trigeminal nerve

posterior spinocerebellar tract

anterior spinocerebellar tract

lateral reticular nucleus

hypoglossal nerve

pyramid (corticospinal tract)

cleidomastoid muscles. The spinal root will probably not be present on the brain specimen.

Lesions restricted to the central portions of the accessory nerve are rare. They are usually included in more global pathology involving the vagus and glossopharyngeal nerves. In any case, destruction of the central motor nuclei or the peripheral nerve results in paresis or paralysis of the two innervated muscles. Elevation and outward rotation of the arm will then be accomplished with difficulty.

The *hypoglossal nerve* (CN XII) arises from the motor neurons of the *hypoglossal nucleus,* the rostral portion of which is located beneath the hypoglossal trigone in the floor of the fourth ventricle. The nucleus continues caudally near the midline throughout the central gray of the closed portion of the medulla (Figs. 10-7 to 10-10). The fibers from this nucleus pass ventrally through the medulla and leave it in a series of 10 or more rootlets along the *ventrolateral sulcus,* between the pyramid and the olive (Fig. 10-1). These rootlets fuse and, as the hypoglossal nerve, leave the cranial cavity through the hypoglossal canal. Extracranially, these fibers are distributed to the ipsilateral intrinsic muscles of the tongue and to the extrinsic muscles (styloglossus, hypoglossus, and genioglossus), which they innervate.

Lesions of the hypoglossal nucleus will result in paresis or paralysis of the muscles of the tongue on the ipsilateral side. The affected side becomes flaccid. Because of the paralysis of the genioglossus muscle, attempts to protrude the tongue result in deviation of the tongue to the side of the lesion due to the greater force of this muscle on the contralateral side.

The dorsal (posterior) surface of the medulla is partially hidden by the overlying cerebellum. By exerting gentle downward pressure on the medulla it is possible to examine more of its surface. The pia and arachnoid adhere tightly to the surface of the medulla. A clearer view such as that shown in Figure 11-4 can be obtained by stripping away the attached meninges and blood vessels from this surface with fine forceps. The dorsal surface of the medulla is divided into an *open* portion and a *closed* portion. The former contains the caudal one-half of the fourth ventricle, which will be examined in detail in the next chapter. The latter encloses the rostral extension of the central canal of the spinal cord. The point at which the open and closed portions meet in the midline at the cranial end of the dorsal median sulcus is known as the *obex* (Fig. 11-4).

The medial *fasciculus gracilis* and the lateral *fasiculus cuneatus* of the spinal cord continue rostrally into the medulla on each side of the *dorsal median sulcus,* as they are in the cervical and upper thoracic segments of the spinal cord. These fasciculi consist of large myelinated fibers conveying impulses concerned with proprioception (position and movement), discriminative touch, pressure, and vibration. Nerve impulses from the appropriate sensory receptors in the lower half of the body are conveyed in the fasciculus gracilis, and from the upper half of the body in the fasciculus cuneatus. The swelling at the upper end of the fasciculus gracilis is the *gracile tubercle,* formed by the underlying *nucleus gracilis.* It is here that the axons of the first neurons of the fasciculus gracilis terminate. Similarly, the swelling at the rostral end of the fasciculus cuneatus is the *cuneate tubercle,* formed by the subjacent *nucleus cuneatus* (Figs. 10-10 and 10-11; see also Fig. 11-4) and fibers of the fasciculus cuneatus terminate in this nucleus. The medial lemniscus takes its origin from these nuclei; the axons of second order neurons (*internal arcuate fibers*) cross to the opposite side in the *decussation of the medial lemniscus* (Fig. 10-10). The medial lemniscus ascends through the brain stem to terminate in the ventral posterior nucleus of the thalamus. From here fibers are relayed via the thalamic radiation of the internal capsule to the postcentral gyrus of the cerebral cortex.

Finally, the transverse fibers of the basilar pons and the course of the corticospinal fibers throughout the brain stem may now be demonstrated. Clear away all the meninges and blood vessels from the ventral (anterior) surface of the brain stem from its transection at the midbrain–diencephalic junction to the caudal medulla. Make a longitudinal midline incision in the basilar pons from the interpeduncular fossa to the bulbopontine sulcus with the blade of the scalpel. This incision should not be more than 2 mm deep. Grasp the cut edge with fine forceps and tear the tissue of the basilar pons laterally toward the middle cerebellar peduncle and the root of the trigeminal nerve. The transverse pontocerebellar fibers are thus easily seen. This should be done on one side only throughout the length

Figure 10-11. Weigert-stained transverse section through the medulla oblongata at the level of the decussation of the pyramids. The solid black line in the key photograph shows the precise plane at which the section was taken.

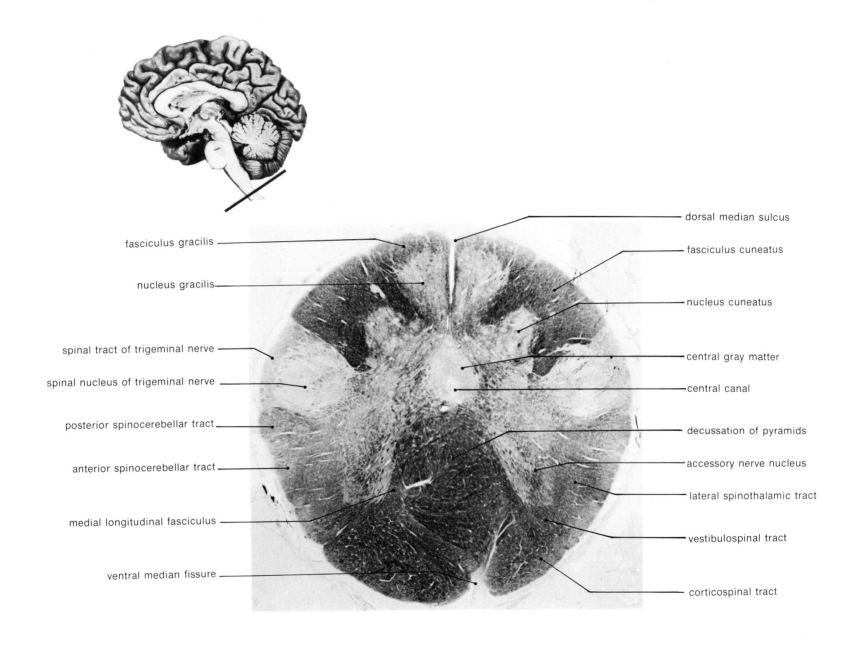

dorsal median sulcus

fasciculus gracilis

nucleus gracilis

fasciculus cuneatus

nucleus cuneatus

spinal tract of trigeminal nerve

spinal nucleus of trigeminal nerve

central gray matter

central canal

posterior spinocerebellar tract

decussation of pyramids

anterior spinocerebellar tract

accessory nerve nucleus

lateral spinothalamic tract

medial longitudinal fasciculus

vestibulospinal tract

ventral median fissure

corticospinal tract

97

of the pons. The other side is left intact in order to compare the internal structure with the external features. The result should look like the dissection shown in Figure 10-12a. Now make a transverse incision across the medullary pyramid on the same side about 1 cm caudal to the bulbopontine sulcus. This incision also should not be more than 2 mm deep. With large forceps grasp the corticospinal fibers contained within the pyramid proximal to the incision and tear

them rostrally (see Fig. 10-12b). The course of these fibers through the pons to the basis pedunculi of the midbrain will be seen easily. Now grasp the fibers distal to the incision in the pyramid and tear them caudally (see Fig. 10-12c). You will notice the vast majority of these fibers crossing to the opposite side at the decussation of the pyramids. The final dissection should look similar to that shown in Figure 10-12d.

Figure 10-12. Dissection of the ventral (anterior) surface of the brain stem to disclose the transverse and longitudinal fibers: (a) Transverse pontocerebellar fibers in the right basilar pons. The left side remains intact. (b) Tearing the corticospinal fibers of the right pyramid rostrally through the pons to the basis pedunculi. (c) Tearing the corticospinal fibers of the right pyramid caudally toward the decussation of the pyramids. (d) The completed dissection showing the course of the corticospinal fibers from midbrain to medullary pyramid.

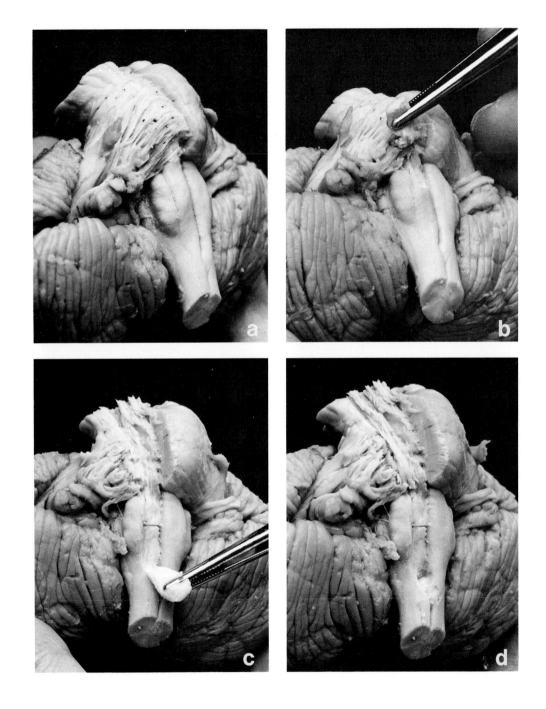

11

Cerebellum and Fourth Ventricle

It has been said that the cerebellum is that part of the brain that is concerned solely with somatic motor activity. In light of recent investigations, such a restricted functional definition of the cerebellum is no longer tenable. This part of the central nervous system plays a major role in the synergism of smooth motor activity; however, evidence suggests that it may be involved in the initiation of movement and the learning of skilled motor movements as well. Physiological studies have revealed that the cerebellum may also influence several autonomic functions, such as the carotid sinus reflex and the cardiovascular, respiratory, and urinary bladder reflexes. It is not incorrect, therefore, to state that the cerebellum is a part of the brain that may influence most activities of the central nervous system. Even so, this part of the brain is not essential for life. Individuals born with a condition in which much of the cerebellum and the pons fail to develop (neocerebellar agenesis) show no obvious neurologic symptoms. In these cases it is likely that other motor regions of the brain assume the functions of the cerebellum. This assumption is supported by the clinical observation that individuals with slowly progressing cerebellar pathology demonstrate fewer neurologic symptoms than those in whom the pathology is of sudden onset.

For the beginning student of neuroanatomy, the structure of the cerebellum is perhaps more difficult to understand than are its functions. Referring to the embryology of the region often helps in understanding the organization of the adult cerebellum. In the 13-mm embryo, the roof plate covering the rhomboid fourth ventricle is very thin. The cerebellum develops from the alar lamina on each side of this thin roof plate. This part of the alar lamina is called the *rhombic lip.* The anterior part of each rhombic lip grows upward and medially to meet in the midline covering the roof plate just behind the mesencephalon. The lateral parts of this cerebellar rudiment grow rapidly and ultimately form the cerebellar hemispheres. By the time the embryo has reached 120 mm (at the end of the fourth month), fissures begin to appear on the surface of the developing cerebellum. The first to develop is the *dorsolateral (posterolateral) fissure,* which separates the most caudal part of the cerebellum from the rest both laterally and in the midline. This caudal part is composed of the *nodule,* in the midline, and the two lateral *flocculi;* together they form the *flocculonodular lobe or lobule.* This lobule is phylogenetically and ontogenetically the oldest part of the cerebellum. The remainder of the cerebellum undergoes massive growth upward, forward, and backward to such an extent that in the adult the dorsolateral fissure becomes displaced to a ventral position.

Now examine the specimen containing the brain stem and the cerebellum, which was separated from the rest of the brain in Chapter 6. Notice the tent-shaped appearance of the dorsal surface of the cerebellum, that is, elevated in the midline and extending laterally as two shallow, sloping concavities. This shape conforms to that of the tentorium cerebelli, to which this surface is closely apposed in life. By contrast, the ventral surface is formed of two bulging con-

Figure 11-1. View of the superior surface of the cerebellum.

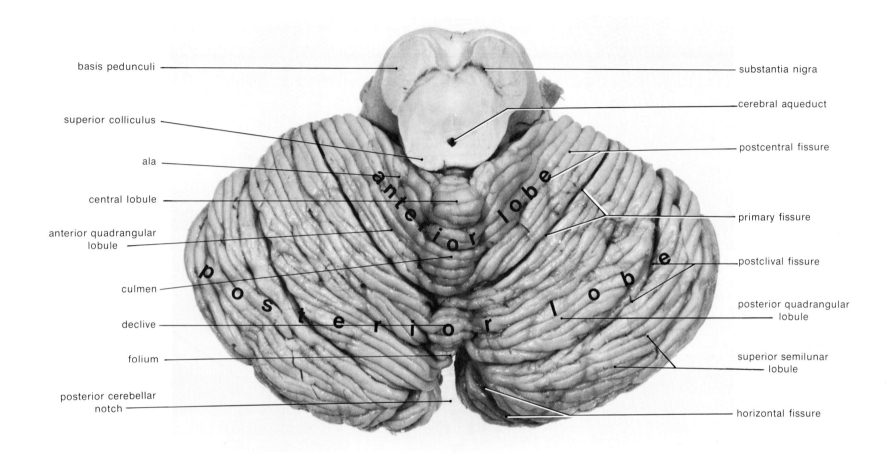

basis pedunculi

superior colliculus

ala

central lobule

anterior quadrangular
lobule

culmen

declive

folium

posterior cerebellar
notch

substantia nigra

cerebral aqueduct

postcentral fissure

primary fissure

postclival fissure

posterior quadrangular
lobule

superior semilunar
lobule

horizontal fissure

anterior lobe

posterior lobe

vexities of neural tissue, one on each side of the brain stem. In the midline, the posterior and inferior surfaces contain a wide and deep groove known as the *vallecula*. That portion of the cerebellum located in the midline on both the dorsal and the ventral surfaces is called the *vermis*. The remainder is the *corpus cerebelli,* which is composed of two large *cerebellar hemispheres.* That portion of the hemisphere located immediately adjacent to the vermis although not demarcated by any sulcus or fissure is known as the *paravermal area.* The surface of the cerebellum is thrown into many convolutions, which are called *cerebellar folia* because of their small size and leaflike appearance.

Anatomically, the cerebellum is divisible into several lobes by sulci and fissures that are for the most part arranged horizontally or transversely. The first fissure to appear, the *dorsolateral fissure,* has been described already. Because of the mushroomlike growth of the corpus cerebelli, this fissure comes to lie on the ventral surface in the adult. Turn the specimen so that the ventral surface faces you. The deep fissure projecting laterally on each side from about the midregion of the olive is the dorsolateral fissure. Just anterior to this fissure the small flocculi are seen projecting laterally for a distance of about 2 cm on each side of the medulla (Fig. 11-2). The nodule cannot be seen at this stage of the dissection.

The second fisssure to develop does so in the anterior part of the cerebellar primordium within both the vermis and the hemispheres. This is the *primary or preclival fissure;* it is a deep V-shaped fissure on the dorsal surface, with the apex of the V directed caudally about 2.5 cm from the most rostral limit of the superior vermis (Figs. 11-1 and 11-3). That portion of the cerebellum located anterior to the limbs of the primary fissure is called the *anterior lobe.* It in turn is divided by a smaller fissure, the *postcentral fissure,* into an anterior portion, the *ala,* and a posterior portion, the *anterior quadrangular lobule.* The rest of the cerebellum on both the superior and inferior surfaces is the *posterior lobe.* The dorsal surface of the posterior lobe is separated from the ventral surface by the *horizontal fissure.* This fissure begins at the posterior incisure and extends horizontally in a large arc around the hemisphere to meet the dorsolateral fissure.

A better view of the ventral surface of the cerebellum is obtained if it is removed from its attachment to the brain stem. This is accomplished by transecting the three cerebellar peduncles, the *superior, middle,* and *inferior cerebellar peduncles.* The superior peduncles are

hidden from view by the overlying anterior lobe of the cerebellum. With the scalpel handle, dissect away the most rostral part of the anterior lobe on the dorsal surface to expose the underlying superior peduncles. They are two robust columns about a centimeter each in width that project forward from the medullary center of the cerebellum and disappear into the midbrain just behind the inferior colliculi (Fig. 11-4). They are joined across the midline by a thin sheet of white matter forming the roof of the anterior part of the fourth ventricle, the *superior medullary velum* (Fig. 11-4). Attached to the dorsal surface of the superior medullary velum is a thin lamina of vermal cortex known as the *lingula* (Fig. 11-3).

The middle cerebellar peduncles ascend from the dorsolateral aspect of the pons. They are identified by the attachment of the large trigeminal nerve roots that emerge from the surface at the junction of the pons and the middle peduncle. Much of this peduncle is also hidden by the lateral parts of the anterior lobe. Dissect the anterior lobe folia for a short distance distal to the trigeminal nerve roots to expose more of the middle peduncle. It is the largest of the three peduncles.

The inferior peduncle is more difficult to locate. It is formed on the dorsolateral aspect of the medulla and upon reaching the pontocerebellar angle it curves sharply upward into the cerebellum on the medial aspect of the middle peduncle (Fig. 11-4).

Transect the superior cerebellar peduncle by making an incision from the depression between the superior and middle peduncles to the dorsal midline. Repeat the procedure on the opposite side. Transect the middle peduncles about a centimeter above the attachment of the trigeminal nerves. Cut the inferior peduncles from the pontocerebellar angle on each side to meet the incisions made across the middle peduncles. Gently pry the cerebellum away from the brain stem, cutting any attached meninges in the process. Notice that the choroid plexus is attached to the inferior surface of the cerebellar vermis, forming the roof of the fourth ventricle. Set the brain stem thus separated aside for subsequent study of the fourth ventricle.

Now examine the topography of the inferior surface of the cerebellum. The vermis is more conspicuous than its counterpart dorsally and is clearly demarcated from the convex inferior cerebellar

Figure 11-2. Ventral posterior view of the cerebellum with the brain stem attached.

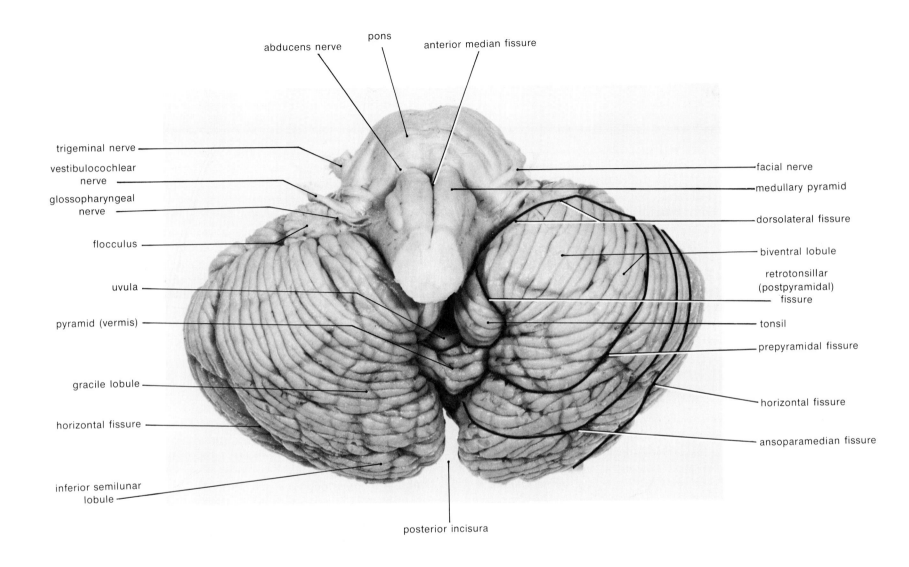

abducens nerve   pons   anterior median fissure

trigeminal nerve

vestibulocochlear
nerve

glossopharyngeal
nerve

flocculus

uvula

pyramid (vermis)

gracile lobule

horizontal fissure

inferior semilunar
lobule

facial nerve

medullary pyramid

dorsolateral fissure

biventral lobule

retrotonsillar
(postpyramidal)
fissure

tonsil

prepyramidal fissure

horizontal fissure

ansoparamedian fissure

posterior incisura

hemispheres by two deep sulci. The most anterior part of the inferior vermis is the *nodule* or nodulus. It is separated from the *uvula* behind by the posterolateral fissure. The midline uvula is connected to a small part of the hemisphere on each side of the vallecula called the *tonsil* (Figs. 11-2 and 11-3).

Like the cerebrum, the cerebellum is constructed of a surface cortical layer of gray matter and a subcortical medullary center composed of myelinated axons. Unlike the cerebral cortex, however, the cerebellar cortex has a constant histological structure throughout. It is composed of three distinct layers: the *molecular layer,* the *Purkinje cell layer,* and the *granular cell layer.*

There are four pairs of nuclei embedded within the medullary center of the cerebellum. The most lateral and the largest is the *dentate nucleus.* Before examining them in your own brain specimen, locate these nuclei in the brain sections shown in Figures 13-3, 13-23, 13-24, 13-41, 13-42, 13-59, and 13-60. With the brain knife make a midline longitudinal cut in the superior vermis not more than 2 cm deep. Now remove successive horizontal slices, each about 5 mm thick and roughly parallel with the superior surface of the hemisphere, through the **right hemisphere.** The elliptical mass of gray matter about 1.5 cm wide and 2.0 cm long located slightly medial to the center of the white matter is the dentate nucleus. It is composed of an irregularly folded lamina of cells, with a central hilus directed forward and medially through which pass the axons of the dentate neurons. These axons form the largest component of the superior cerebellar peduncle. Now make a series of parasagittal sections, each about 5 mm thick, through the **left hemisphere.** On the cut surface of the slices note the characteristic branched pattern of the white matter called the *arbor vitae.* As the slices approach the sagittal plane, the dentate nucleus will be seen again embedded within the white matter of the hemisphere. Three other bilateral pairs of nuclei are located medial to the dentate nucleus, but they are difficult to identify because of their small size. They are the *emboliform, globose,* and *fastigial nuclei.*

Nowhere is the phylogenetic progression in the development of the central nervous system more evident than within the cerebellum. In humans, this is represented by longitudinal divisions of the cerebellum that are based on functional rather than gross anatomic considerations. These divisions are determined largely on the basis of the afferent connections to each. The most medial division, and the

oldest phylogenetically, is known as the *archicerebellum.* It is composed of the paired flocculi and the nodule *(flocculonodular lobule)* together with a portion of the adjoining *uvula* of the inferior vermis. This portion receives afferent fibers from the vestibular apparatus of the inner ear, both direct fibers from the vestibular ganglion, and indirect fibers from the vestibular nuclei of the medulla via the inferior cerebellar peduncle. The Purkinje cell axons of the archicerebellar cortex project largely to the fastigial nucleus. This nucleus in turn projects axons to the four vestibular nuclei of the medulla, from which arise the vestibulospinal tracts and the medial longitudinal fasciculus. The archicerebellum, therefore, is associated with the maintenance of muscle tone in response to vestibular stimulation and functions in maintaining equilibrium and balance. For this reason the archicerebellum is also known as the *vestibulocerebellum.*

The superior vermis of the anterior lobe as well as the inferior vermis (with the exception of the nodule and to some extent the uvula) are known collectively as the *paleocerebellum.* This region, along with the neighboring medial parts of each hemisphere, receives its afferent fibers directly from the dorsal spinocerebellar tract via the inferior peduncle and from the ventral spinocerebellar tract, which enters the cerebellum as a component of the superior peduncle. In addition, it receives indirect projections from the spinal cord by way of the dorsal and ventral accessory olivary nuclei and the accessory cuneate nucleus; the axons of the neurons of the latter nuclei enter the cerebellum via the inferior peduncle. Fibers from the chief sensory and spinal nuclei of the trigeminal complex and from the lateral reticular nucleus also reach the paleocerebellum. The Purkinje cells of the paleocerebellar cortex project to the globose and emboliform (and to some degree to the fastigial) nuclei. The axons of these neurons in turn terminate largely in the red nucleus and the nuclei of the reticular formation. The paleocerebellum therefore serves to coordinate the musculature of the trunk and of the limbs for the maintenance of posture in response to sensory input from cutaneous exteroceptors and muscle, joint, and tendon proprioceptors. It is thus also known as the *spinocerebellum.*

The most lateral of the three divisions is called the *neocerebellum,*

Figure 11-3. Medial view of the right half of the cerebellum with attached brain stem. Structures in the midline of the cerebellar vermis are demonstrated.

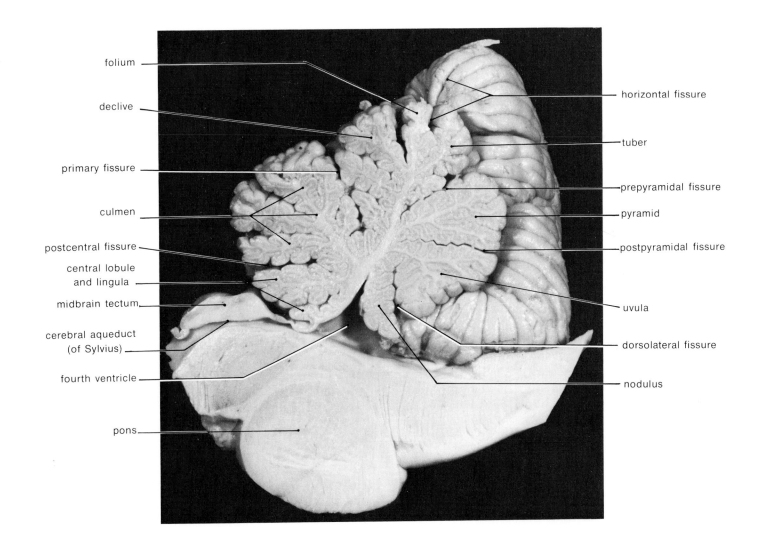

folium

declive

primary fissure

culmen

postcentral fissure

central lobule
and lingula

midbrain tectum

cerebral aqueduct
(of Sylvius)

fourth ventricle

pons

horizontal fissure

tuber

prepyramidal fissure

pyramid

postpyramidal fissure

uvula

dorsolateral fissure

nodulus

105

because it is the most recent acquisition phylogenetically. It is composed of the lateral parts of the cerebellar hemispheres, including the superior vermis of the posterior lobe. It is found only in mammals in conjunction with the appearance of the neocortex of the cerebral hemispheres and the ventrolateral nuclei of the thalamus. It receives large numbers of afferents from the cerebral cortex, none of which is direct. The most massive projection is from the sensorimotor cortex to the ipsilateral pontine nuclei, which in turn project largely to the contralateral cerebellar hemisphere via the middle cerebellar peduncle. This is the *corticopontocerebellar pathway,* and it is because of this that the neocerebellum is often referred to as the *pontocerebellum.* In addition to this pathway, the inferior olivary nucleus, which receives projection fibers from the motor cortex among other sources, projects in a topographic fashion to the contralateral cerebellar hemisphere via the inferior peduncle. The Purkinje cells of the hemisphere project to the dentate nucleus. The axons of neurons in this latter nucleus form the largest component of the superior cerebellar peduncle and terminate in the contralateral ventral lateral thalamic nucleus. The thalamic nucleus in turn projects to the motor and premotor cortex, thus completing the circuit. This closed neuroanatomic circuit suggests that the neocerebellum exerts a controlling or modulating influence over the motor activity of the neocortex, especially with respect to the distal musculature of the limbs. Lesions of the neocerebellum result in asynergy and decomposition of muscular movement and in intention tremor which is most evident in the upper limb of the ipsilateral side.

Cerebellar control and coordination of motor activity is totally ipsilateral. Although there may be decussations in both the afferent and the efferent pathways of the cerebellum, the presence of compensating decussations ensures that the motor influences are ultimately ipsilateral.

Fourth Ventricle

When viewed from the sagittal plane the roof of the fourth ventricle is a tent-shaped cavity, with the apex of the cavity directed upward into the cerebellum (Fig. 11-3). Removal of the cerebellum from the brain stem, as has already been accomplished, provides an unobstructed view of the floor of this ventricle, which is called the *rhomboid fossa* because of its four-sided, diamond-shaped appearance (Fig.

11-4). The rostral point of the ventricle is continuous with the narrow *cerebral aqueduct (of Sylvius)* as it emerges from the midbrain; at its caudal limit the ventricle is continuous with the central canal of the medulla and the spinal cord.

A better understanding of the structures found within the floor of the rhomboid fossa is gained if one considers the developmental origin of this region. Early in its development, for example, by the end of the first month (11-mm embryo), the neural tube consists of masses of cells that form the thick lateral walls of the tube. The roof plate and the floor plate are relatively thin. A shallow groove, the *sulcus limitans,* indents the thick lateral walls longitudinally to separate the *alar lamina* of cells above the sulcus from the *basal lamina* of cells below the sulcus. The alar lamina moves laterally, causing the roof plate to become stretched and attenuated. This lateral movement is carried to such an extent that the sulcus limitans, which once was located on the lateral wall of the neural tube, now comes to lie on the floor of the expanded diamond-shaped cavity (Fig. 11-4). It therefore follows that the cranial nerve nuclei that will ultimately develop from the alar lamina of cells, now lateral to the sulcus limitans, will be afferent (sensory) in function, while those developing medial to the sulcus limitans will be efferent (motor) in function.

Now examine the floor of the fourth ventricle in the specimen. In the midline lies a longitudinal sulcus, the *median sulcus* (Fig. 11-4), which divides the floor into symmetrical right and left halves. On each side of the median sulcus there is an elevated ridge; this is the *median eminence* of the fourth ventricle, beneath which lies the motor nuclei of some of the cranial nerves. In the anterior part of the ventricle the median eminence is wide, forming almost the entire floor of the ventricle. Midway between the median sulcus and the lateral edges of the ventricle, a shallow curved groove, the *sulcus limitans,* may be seen running longitudinally. Halfway in its longitudinal course it widens to form a small dimple, the *superior fovea.* That portion of the median eminence located between the superior fovea and the median sulcus is the *facial colliculus.* The elevation in the floor is caused

---

Figure 11-4. Dorsal (posterior) surface of the brain stem following removal of the cerebellum by transection of the superior, middle, and inferior cerebellar peduncles. This procedure provides an unobstructed view of the structures on the floor of the fourth ventricle.

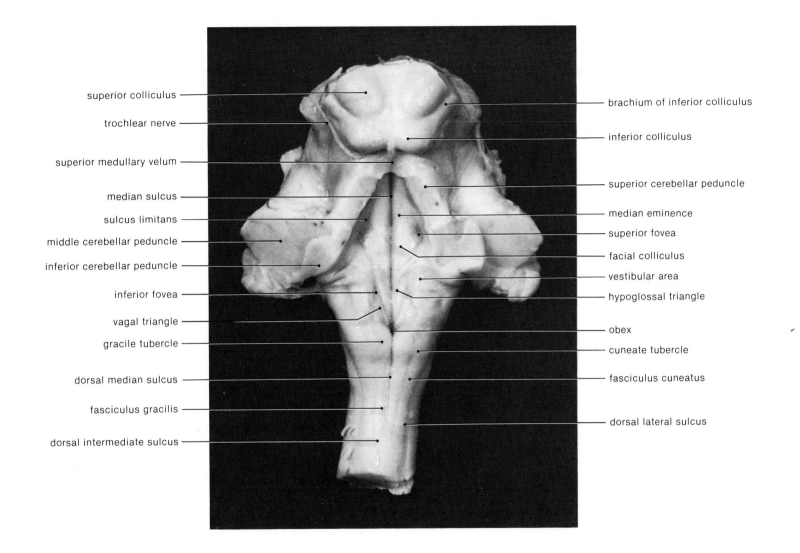

superior colliculus

trochlear nerve

superior medullary velum

median sulcus

sulcus limitans

middle cerebellar peduncle

inferior cerebellar peduncle

inferior fovea

vagal triangle

gracile tubercle

dorsal median sulcus

fasciculus gracilis

dorsal intermediate sulcus

brachium of inferior colliculus

inferior colliculus

superior cerebellar peduncle

median eminence

superior fovea

facial colliculus

vestibular area

hypoglossal triangle

obex

cuneate tubercle

fasciculus cuneatus

dorsal lateral sulcus

by the underlying internal genu of the facial nerve looping around and over the abducens nucleus, which is located here. Within the floor of the fourth ventricle at the level of the rostral pons, identify an area in the sulcus limitans that is faintly bluish-black in color. This is the *locus ceruleus,* an important noradrenergic center of the brain. It derives its name from the constituent neurons, which contain a melanin pigment that gives the area its characteristic appearance. The area of the ventricle located lateral to the sulcus limitans contains the sensory nuclei of the cranial nerves.

Identify a number of horizontal bands of fibers running transversely across the floor of the ventricle; these are the *striae medullares* of the fourth ventricle. They may not be too obvious in some specimens. These fibers arise from neurons of the arcuate nucleus, which is situated just lateral to the pyramids of the medulla (Fig. 10-10). The axons run dorsally in the midline and then curve laterally on the floor of the ventricle to enter the cerebellum by way of the inferior cerebellar peduncle. The striae medullares conveniently divide the floor of the ventricle into rostral and caudal halves.

In the caudal half of the ventricle, the sulcus limitans widens again to form another small dimple; this is the *inferior fovea.* Lateral to the inferior fovea and extending rostrally under the striae medullares is the *vestibular area,* beneath which lies the complex of vestibular nuclei. Behind the striae medullares near the midline there are two small triangular elevations, one on each side of the median sulcus. These are the *hypoglossal triangles,* beneath which are located the *nuclei of the hypoglossal nerves.* Lateral and caudal to the hypoglossal triangles and behind the inferior foveae are the *vagal triangles,* beneath which are the *dorsal nuclei of the vagus nerve.* In some specimens a very fine ridge may be seen diagonally traversing the vagal triangle. This is the *funiculus separans.* Between this ridge and the gracile tubercle lies a small area known as the *area postrema.* This area, similar to several other midline structures of the ventricular system, is devoid of a blood–brain barrier. Because the caudal floor of the fourth ventricle bears a resemblance to the nib of a pen, it is sometimes called the *calamus scriptorius.*

Finally make a series of transverse slices, each about 0.5 cm thick, through what is left of the brain stem beginning at the level of the superior colliculus. Examine the cut surface of each successive slice. Even in the unstained preparation, you should be able to identify some of the larger and more prominent brain stem structures described in this and the previous chapter.

12

Spinal Cord

The spinal cord is an elongated, almost cylindrical, structure that occupies the *vertebral canal* of the spine, or vertebral column. In the adult, the spinal cord is about 42–45 cm long and occupies only the upper two-thirds of the vertebral canal. It extends from the foramen magnum, where it is continuous with the medulla oblongata, to the level of the intervertebral disk between the first and second lumbar vertebrae.

In the specimen of spinal cord provided for this laboratory, first examine the investing meninges. The outermost of the meningeal layers is the *dura mater*. The spinal dura is a long tubular sleeve of thick fibrous connective tissue that completely encloses the cord. It extends from the foramen magnum to the level of the second sacral vertebra. At the foramen magnum the spinal dura is attached to the occipital bone of the skull and is continuous with the cranial dura, which encloses the brain. At the level of the second sacral vertebra, the spinal dura continues as part of the *filum terminale* (Fig. 12-1), a slender filamentous extension of the spinal cord of unknown functional significance. The filum with its dural investment extends beyond the second sacral vertebra as the coccygeal ligament to become attached to the dorsum of the coccyx. The spinal dura, unlike its cranial counterpart, is separated from the bony walls of the vertebral canal by a space called the *epidural space*. This space contains fat, loose connective tissue, and a plexus of veins—the *internal vertebral venous plexus*. In addition, the spinal dura is not reflected to form septa and does not enclose venous sinuses, as does the cranial dura. Observe the sleeves of dura that invest the spinal nerve roots and

ganglia. Distally, these sleeves are attached to the periosteum of the vertebrae at the intervertebral foramina.

The spinal *arachnoid* is a delicate translucent membrane continuous with and not unlike its counterpart investing the brain. Normally it is closely adherent to the inner surface of the spinal dura and conforms to it in both shape and size. It along with the dural sleeve ends in a cul-de-sac below the level of the second sacral vertebrae. The spinal *subarachnoid space* occupies the interval between the arachnoid and the innermost meningeal layer, the *pia mater*. In life this space is filled with cerebrospinal fluid and is continuous with the cranial subarachnoid space. Below the second lumbr vertebra the subarachnoid space is especially large and contains the nerve roots of the *cauda equina*. This space is known as the *lumbar cistern*. It exists because the length of the vertebral canal exceeds that of the spinal cord in the adult. The spinal cord ends at the lower border of the first lumbar vertebra, and the lumbar cistern extends from this level to the lower border of the second sacral vertebra. Clinical advantage is often taken of this enlarged subarachnoid space to obtain samples of cerebrospinal fluid by lumbar puncture or spinal tap without risk of injury to the spinal cord.

The *pia mater* is a delicate membrane that adheres tightly to the substance of the spinal cord and encloses the blood vessels of the cord. In the specimen provided, the meninges described above should be incised and pinned laterally. Notice a longitudinal band of pia mater on each side of the cord. These bands extend laterally from each side midway between the dorsal and the ventral roots. These

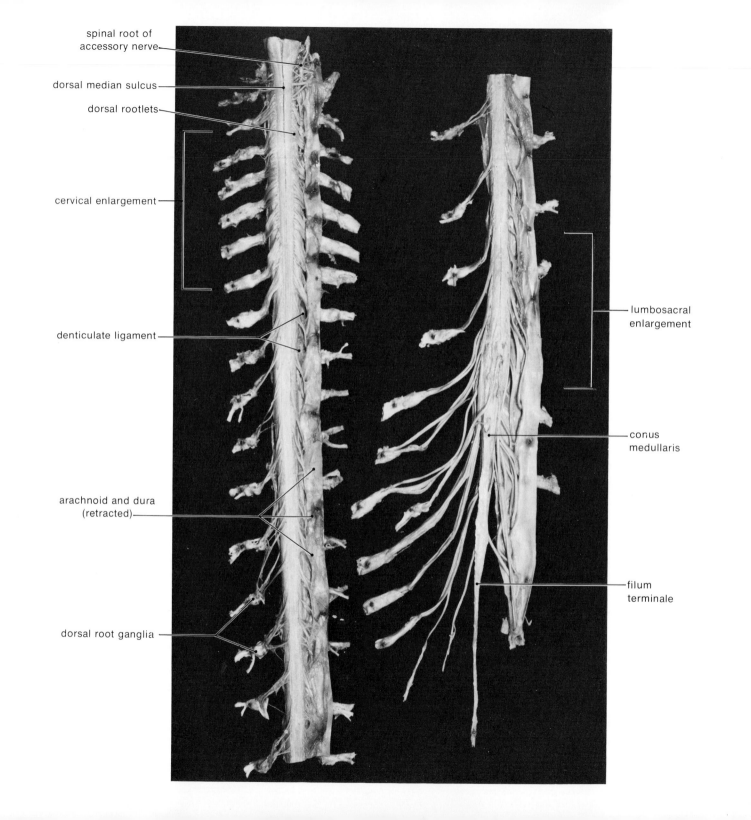

spinal root of
accessory nerve

dorsal median sulcus

dorsal rootlets

cervical enlargement

denticulate ligament

arachnoid and dura
(retracted)

dorsal root ganglia

lumbosacral
enlargement

conus
medullaris

filum
terminale

are the *denticulate ligaments*, which serve to suspend the spinal cord within the dural sheath (Figs. 12-1 and 12-2). At 21 pairs of points along the length of the cord, this pial sheath pierces the arachnoid and inserts into the dura. Identify some of these points of insertion in your spinal cord specimen. The pia mater extends beyond the tapered conical end of the spinal cord *(conus medullaris)* as part of the filum terminale. The *filum terminale* consists mainly of pia mater, although neuroglia are present for part of its length. As already stated, the filum pierces both the arachnoid and the dura at the level of the second sacral vertebra; it receives an investment from both of these layers and continues to the coccyx as the coccygeal ligament.

Before studying the spinal cord itself, identify as much of the blood supply of the spinal cord as you can on the specimen. You will recall from Chapter 5 that the arterial blood supply of the cord is derived from spinal branches of the *vertebral arteries* and from *segmental vessels* (cervical, intercostal, lumbar, and sacral). A single *anterior spinal artery* descends within the ventral median fissure, and two *posterior spinal* arteries descend along the line of attachment of the dorsal roots. These spinal arteries are reinforced along the length of the cord by a variable number of *radicular arteries,* which are branches of segmental vessels. These arteries traverse the intervertebral foramina, divide into anterior and posterior branches, and contribute to a longitudinal anastomotic network of channels encircling the cord. Small branches from the anterior spinal artery supply the gray matter of the ventral (anterior) columns to the base of the dorsal (posterior) columns and the white matter of the adjacent funiculi. The posterior spinal arteries and their branches supply the remainder of the dorsal gray columns and the white matter of the dorsal funiculi. The veins of the spinal cord have a distribution similar to that of the arteries. They usually drain into six longitudinal venous channels at the surface of the cord. This irregular plexus of veins communicates freely with the internal vertebral venous plexus located within the epidural space and with segmental veins via a series of radicular veins. These latter veins will not be present in the specimen.

Now direct your attention to the spinal cord itself. Note that it is not of uniform diameter throughout its length; it is largest at cervical levels and smallest at sacral levels. In two locations, between C4 and T1 and between L1 and S2, the cord is noticeably enlarged. The former is the *cervical enlargement,* which gives rise to the nerves that innervate the upper limb; the latter is the *lumbosacral enlargement,* which gives rise to nerves that innervate the lower limb (Figs. 12-1 and 12-3). Furthermore, the cord is not entirely cylindrical in shape; rather, its width exceeds its dorsoventral dimension. This is most evident in the region of the cervical enlargement (Fig. 12-3). Examine the dorsal and ventral surfaces of the cord. Note that it is marked by a midline longitudinal furrow on both surfaces. The one on the ventral or anterior surface is the *ventral median fissure.* It is deeper than its counterpart on the dorsal or posterior surface, the *dorsal median sulcus.* Some idea of the depth of the ventral median fissure is obtained by incising the meninges in the midline in the region of the cervical enlargement and inserting a blunt probe into the fissure.

Externally, the cord has a segmented appearance due to the series of paired spinal nerves that arise from it. It must be emphasized, however, that internally the cord is not segmented; it is composed of a continuum of columns of gray and white matter. Thirty-one pairs of spinal nerves arise from the cord, each of which is attached to the cord by a *ventral (motor) root* and a usually larger *dorsal (sensory) root.* Close to the cord these roots break up into a series of smaller rootlets (Fig. 12-2). Eight pairs of cervical, 12 pairs of thoracic, 5 pairs of lumbar, 5 pairs of sacral, and 1 pair of coccygeal spinal nerves can usually be distinguished. In a small percentage of humans the dorsal roots of the first pair of cervical nerves may be absent. As mentioned earlier, each dorsal root is attached to the cord by a series of rootlets. Their attachment to the cord is along a shallow longitudinal depression called the *dorsolateral sulcus* (Figs. 12-2 and 12-3). Similarly, each ventral root emerges from the cord as a series of rootlets from a less distinct line called the *ventrolateral sulcus.* Above midthoracic levels, an additional longitudinal sulcus may be identified between the dorsal median and the dorsolateral sulci. This is the *dorsal intermediate sulcus.* Each of the dorsal roots possesses a prominent enlargement, *the dorsal root ganglion,* which contains the cell bodies of afferent neurons that enter the spinal cord. The dorsal root ganglia are located in the intervertebral foramina except the first two cervical, which are on the vertebral arches of the atlas and axis and those of the sacral and coccygeal nerves, which are in the

Figure 12-1. The spinal cord viewed from its dorsal surface. The meninges have been removed from the left half and retracted on the right half of the specimen. The cord has been cut at the junction between segments T10 and T11.

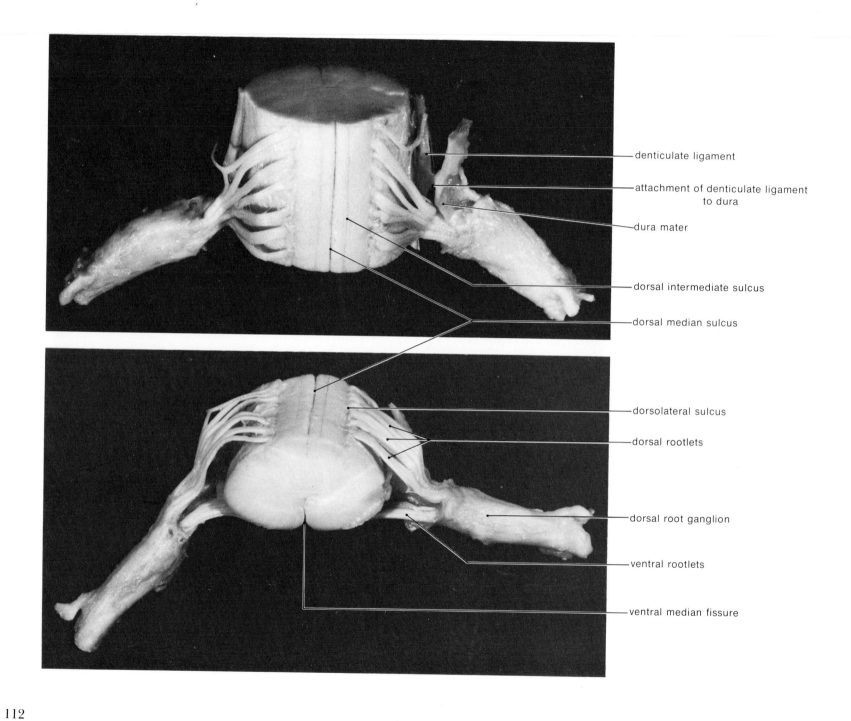

denticulate ligament

attachment of denticulate ligament
to dura

dura mater

dorsal intermediate sulcus

dorsal median sulcus

dorsolateral sulcus

dorsal rootlets

dorsal root ganglion

ventral rootlets

ventral median fissure

112

vertebral canal and dura, respectively. The dorsal and ventral roots unite immediately distal to the ganglion to form spinal nerves that emerge from the intervertebral foramina.

Carefully trace the course taken by a pair of dorsal and ventral roots. They traverse the subarachnoid space, pierce the arachnoid and the dura separately, and after traversing the epidural space reach the interveretebral foramina, where the ganglia are located. Note that cervical nerve roots pursue a short, almost horizontal course to their point of exit from the vertebral column. The remaining nerve roots, however, increase successively in both length and obliquity from thoracic to sacral levels en route to their exit from the vertebral column. This is due to the fact that, in the adult, the spinal cord is shorter than the vertebral column. The roots of the lumbosacral and coccygeal nerves are the longest and extend for some distance beyond the conus medullaris of the cord to reach their respective foramina. This collection of the spinal nerve roots in the lower subarachnoid space resembles the hair on a horse's tail and is therefore called the *cauda equina*. These nerve roots are sometimes compressed by herniated intervertebral disks as they traverse the intervertebral foramina. A common site for this to occur is between L4–5 and L5–S1 causing pain of the lower back and possibly of the lower limbs accompanied by reduced cutaneous sensation and muscle weakness within the area supplied by the nerve.

Before proceeding with the internal structure of the cord, students are advised to review with the aid of a textbook illustration or model the anatomic relationship that exists between the spinal cord segments and their corresponding vertebrae. One spinal cord segment comprises that length of cord to which a pair of nerve roots is attached. The location of spinal cord segments relative to their bony vertebral investment is important clinically. In the cervical region the spinous processes of the vertebrae overlie succeeding segments of the spinal cord. In the upper thoracic region the spinous processes overlie cord segments two displaced in number whereas in the lower thoracic region the difference increases to three segments. All of the lumbar segments of the cord lie opposite the spinous processes of

---

Figure 12-2. One segment of the spinal cord showing the entrance of the dorsal rootlets and the emergence of the ventral rootlets, the denticulate ligament, and the dorsal root ganglia.

the tenth to the twelfth thoracic vertebrae. Sacral and coccygeal spinal cord segments are located at the level of the spinous process of the first lumbar vertebra.

Cervical spinal nerves (C1–7) leave the vertebral canal through the intervertebral foramina above their corresponding vertebra numerically. The ventral rami of the first two cervical nerves lie on the vertebral arches of the atlas and axis, respectively. Recall that there are eight cervical nerves but only seven cervical vertebrae. The eighth cervical nerve, therefore, exists between the seventh cervical and the first thoracic vertebrae. All of the remaining spinal nerves, beginning with the first thoracic, leave the vertebral column below their corresponding vertebra numerically.

Many of the features observed in the gross specimen can be identified in the three transverse sections of the spinal cord shown in Figure 12-3. In each of the three illustrations one-half of the section demonstrates the fibers of the white matter and the other half demonstrates the nuclear material of the gray matter of the cord. Identify the dorsal median sulcus, ventral median fissure, dorsolateral sulcus, ventrolateral sulcus, and dorsal intermediate sulcus. Notice also that the cervical and thoracic segments of the cord are flattened dorsoventrally, whereas the lumbosacral segments are almost cylindrical in shape. Notice that the central gray matter is smallest in the thoracic region and largest in the cervical and lumbosacral regions. Why is this? Notice also that the amount of white matter increases considerably from lumbosacral to cervical levels of the cord. Why is this?

The peripheral white matter of the cord is organized into three paired columns of fibers. These columns are called *funiculi*. The *dorsal funiculus* is that portion of white matter located between the dorsal median sulcus and the dorsolateral sulcus. The *lateral funiculus* is that region of white matter located between the dorsal and ventral roots, that is, between the dorsolateral and ventrolateral sulci. The *ventral funiculus* is that region of white matter located between the ventrolateral sulcus and the ventral median fissure (Fig. 12-3). These funiculi contain the many ascending and descending fiber tracts of the cord. Students are advised to review at this point the names and location of the major fiber tracts of the cord: fasciculus cuneatus, fasciculus gracilis, spinothalamic tract, dorsal and ventral spinocerebellar tracts, lateral and anterior corticospinal tracts, and vestibulospinal tract.

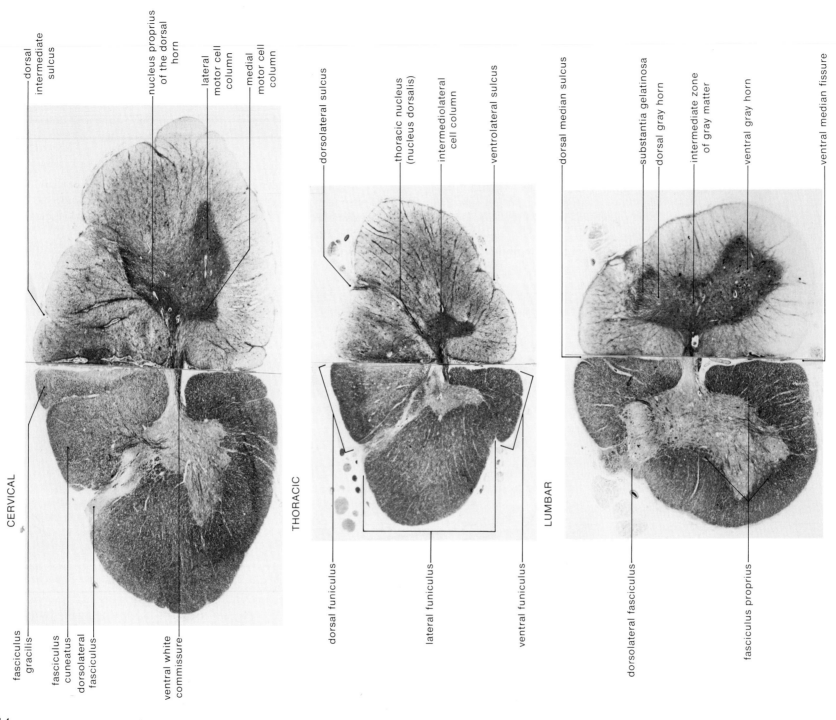

CERVICAL

fasciculus gracilis

dorsal intermediate sulcus

nucleus proprius of the dorsal horn

lateral motor cell column

medial motor cell column

fasciculus cuneatus

dorsolateral fasciculus

ventral white commissure

THORACIC

dorsolateral sulcus

thoracic nucleus (nucleus dorsalis)

intermediolateral cell column

ventrolateral sulcus

dorsal funiculus

lateral funiculus

ventral funiculus

LUMBAR

dorsal median sulcus

substantia gelatinosa

dorsal gray horn

intermediate zone of gray matter

ventral gray horn

ventral median fissure

dorsolateral fasciculus

fasciculus proprius

114

The gray matter of the cord adopts roughly the shape of the letter H in transverse section. The two vertical columns of gray matter on each side extend throughout the length of the cord. They are divided into *ventral (anterior)* and *dorsal (posterior) gray horns* or *columns.* The former do not extend to the surface of the cord. The dorsal and ventral horns are joined in the midline by a horizontal gray commissure. The gray commissure contains a slender *central canal,* which is continuous with the ventricular system of the brain but usually obliterated in places along the length of the cord after the second decade of life. The dorsal and ventral gray horns are composed of columns of neurons or nuclei, some of which extend the length of the cord while others are found only in certain regions of the cord. Students are advised to review at this time the names and location of some of the more important columns of cells (nucleus proprius, substantia gelatinosa, nucleus thoracicus, intermediolateral cell column, ventrolateral, ventromedial, and central motor cell columns) within the gray matter of the cord. In recent years a more precise laminar pattern of organization has been proposed for the different regions of spinal cord gray matter. According to this scheme nine different laminae and a tenth region surrounding the central canal can be distinguished throughout the central gray matter of the cord. Lamina II corresponds to the substantia gelatinosa of traditional nomenclature and the nucleus proprius roughly corresponds to laminae III and IV. Lamina VII corresponds to the intermediate gray zone located between the dorsal and ventral horns and includes the nucleus thoracicus and intermediolateral cell column. The somata of motor neurons are contained in lamina IX.

The *sympathetic or thoracolumbar* division of the autonomic nervous system arises from nerve cell bodies located in the *intermediolateral cell column* of the central gray matter. The intermediolateral cell column is present only in the thoracic and upper two lumbar segments of the spinal cord (T1–L2), hence the name thoracolumbar. A group of cells in a similar location in the sacral cord (S2–4) provides the source of outflow of preganglionic pelvic parasympathetic fibers.

Figure 12-3. Transverse sections through cervical, thoracic, and lumbosacral segments of the spinal cord. The section shown in the left half of each photograph has been stained to demonstrate fibers in the white matter; the section in the right half of each photograph has been stained to demonstrate nuclear material of the gray matter of the cord.

Preganglionic sympathetic fibers arising from the intermediolateral cell column leave the spinal cord in the ventral roots of all thoracic and the upper two lumbar spinal nerves. Once outside the intervertebral foramen, the preganglionic fibers leave the anterior or ventral rami of the peripheral nerves (intercostal nerves in the thoracic region) to join the sympathetic trunk or chain of ganglia via 12 pairs of small communicating trunks called the *white rami communicantes.* The name derives from the fact that preganglionic autonomic fibers are myelinated and fresh myelin has a white appearance.

The *sympathetic trunks* (paravertebral chain of ganglia) are two long columns of interconnected ganglia (nerve cells) located on either side of the vertebral column extending from the upper cervical region to the coccyx. Some preganglionic sympathetic fibers terminate within the sympathetic trunk at the level of entry by synapsing with *ganglion cells.* The axons of these ganglion cells are *nonmyelinated* and referred to as *postganglionic.* They rejoin thoracic spinal nerves via *gray rami communicantes* and are distributed in them to *smooth muscle* and *glands* of the body wall.

Some preganglionic fibers, however, ascend or descend to cervical and lumbosacral regions of the sympathetic trunk before synapsing. Postganglionic fibers leave the sympathetic trunk in these locations as gray rami that join cervical, sacral, and coccygeal spinal nerves. Each of the 31 pairs of spinal nerves, therefore, are joined to the sympathetic trunks by a gray communicating ramus.

Other preganglionic fibers that enter the thoracic part of the sympathetic trunk via white rami communicantes pass through the trunk without synapsing. These myelinated fibers form the following splanchnic nerves: the *greater splanchnic* nerve, arising from the fifth to ninth thoracic sympathetic ganglia, the *lesser splanchnic nerve,* arising from the tenth to eleventh ganglia, and the *least splanchnic* nerve, arising from the twelfth thoracic ganglion, which pierce the diaphragm and innervate the abdominal viscera. *Splanchnic* nerves, therefore, are preganglionic fibers that do not synapse in the sympathetic trunk but in prevertebral ganglia situated in the abdominal cavity.

If prosected specimens of the interior walls of the thorax are provided for this laboratory, identify the anterior or ventral rami of the intercostal nerves, the sympathetic trunk and ganglia, the gray and white rami communicantes, and the splanchnic nerves. Note that all rami communicantes will appear white in these preparations because of their epineurial and perineurial connective tissue investments.

13

Atlas of Brain Sections with C.T. and M.R. Images

The brains used in the preparation of this atlas were fixed for 3 months suspended in 10% formalin by a ligature placed about the basilar artery. Good contrast between gray and white matter in the staining technique is difficult to obtain in brains that have been fixed for periods longer than 3 months. The brains were then washed in running water for 12 hours. If the dura was present on the specimen it was carefully removed. The leptomeninges were left intact for they help to hold the sections together during the slicing procedure. The arachnoid and superficial cerebral blood vessels were removed from the first of the parasagittal and horizontal slices prior to photographing because their presence obstructs the view of the surface morphology of the cortex.

The brain specimens were sectioned on a Berkel rotary meat slicer, (Toronto, Canada) in four different planes: coronal, parasagittal, and two horizontal planes. Each slice was 5 mm thick. Parasagittal sections are obtained easily by starting from the medial surface of a hemisected brain and slicing laterally. However, obtaining accurate slices in the coronal and horizontal planes is more difficult; for slices in these planes meticulous attention was paid to the photographs in the atlas of human brain sections by Matsui and Hirano (1978). This work contains photographs of sections of the brain from 0° to 140° about the canthomeatal line. We chose to use only two horizontal planes; the first was taken parallel to the canthomeatal line (i.e., 0°) and the second was a plane rotated 15° from the canthomeatal line. This latter plane is the one used frequently in computerized tomography of the brain in order to obtain maximum imaging

of subtentorial structures without irradiating the orbit and its contents.

Before each slice was made, the blade and all parts of the slicer over which the brain specimen must slide were lubricated with a solution of 50% glycerine in distilled water.

Each slice was placed on a sheet of white paper in the following manner:

Parasagittal sections were placed with the lateral surface down so that the final view in the photograph would be of the medial surface of each slice.

Coronal slices were placed with the caudal (posterior) surface down so that the final view in the photograph would be of the rostral (anterior) surface of each slice.

Horizontal slices were placed with the inferior surface down so that the final view in the photograph would be of the superior surface of each slice.

An outline of the section was traced in pencil on the paper; the section was removed and the gyri, sulci, and other identifying features were drawn on the paper in rough. The pencilled drawing was immediately labeled with reference to the remainder of the still intact brain. This procedure is important to be able to subsequently identify with certainty all the gyri and sulci on the surface of the cortex in a series of isolated and separate sections without reference to their relationship in the intact brain. The sections were stored for not more than 48 hours in water, separated from each other by paper towels.

Slices of only the surface of the cortex, such as the first parasagittal section showing the medial surface of the hemisphere, were left unstained. In these cases, staining provided no further advantage in the photographic procedure. All other slices were stained with the Le Masurier modification of the Mulligan technique as described by Le Masurier (1935). With this technique, gray matter stains a deep blue color from the Prussian blue reaction whereas the white matter remains relatively unstained. The stained slices were stored in Pulvertaft–Kaiserling mounting fluid III. They were photographed with Ilford FP4 4 × 5 in. sheet film and developed in Ilford Microphen film developer. The final photographs were printed on Ilford Ilfospeed resin-coated paper. The images were enlarged to the same size as the initial pencilled outline of the slice described earlier.

Wherever possible, we have used the more common English nomenclature in labeling the photographs. For this purpose several texts and atlases of the human brain were consulted. They were "An Atlas of the Human Brain for Computerized Tomography" by Matsui and Hirano (1978), "Structure of the Human Brain: A Photographic Atlas" by DeArmond, Fusco, and Dewey (1976), "Neuroanatomy: An Atlas of Structures, Sections and Systems" by Haines (1983), "Atlas of the Central Nervous System in Sectional Planes" by Zuleger and Staubesand (1977), "Atlas of the Central Nervous System in Man" by Miller and Burack (1982), "The Human Nervous System: An Anatomical Viewpoint" by Barr and Kiernan (1983), and "The Human Brain in Dissection," by Montemurro and Bruni (1981, first edition).

For the Latin nomenclature used, our authority has been "Nomina Anatomica," (1977).

Some of the sulci have been accented in the photographs with heavy black lines in one hemisphere only; the other hemisphere was left untouched. Wherever possible, we have labeled surface structures in each section on the right side of the photograph and internal structures on the left. Two key photographs are found at the top of each figure showing the precise plane at which the section was taken. Wherever appropriate, small photographs of computerized tomographs (CT scans) and magnetic resonance (MR) images that correspond as closely as possible to the anatomic section were placed at the bottom of each figure. The CT scans are found at the bottom left and the MR images at the bottom right. These images were taken by Dr. D. Pelz of the Department of Diagnostic Radiology and Nuclear Medicine, University Hospital, London, Ontario, Canada, using normal volunteers. The CT scans were obtained using a GE 9800 unit. The axial, 1-cm-thick slices were taken at approximately 15° to the orbitomeatal baseline. The MR images were obtained using a GE Singa unit operating at 1.5 Tesla. The axial images were obtained using the spin-echo technique with a TR of 2000 msec and TE of 70 msec. Those slices are 0.5 cm thick and were obtained at approximately 0° and 15° to the orbitomeatal baseline. The sagittal images were produced using the partial saturation technique, TR 600 msec and TE 20 msec.

MIDLINE

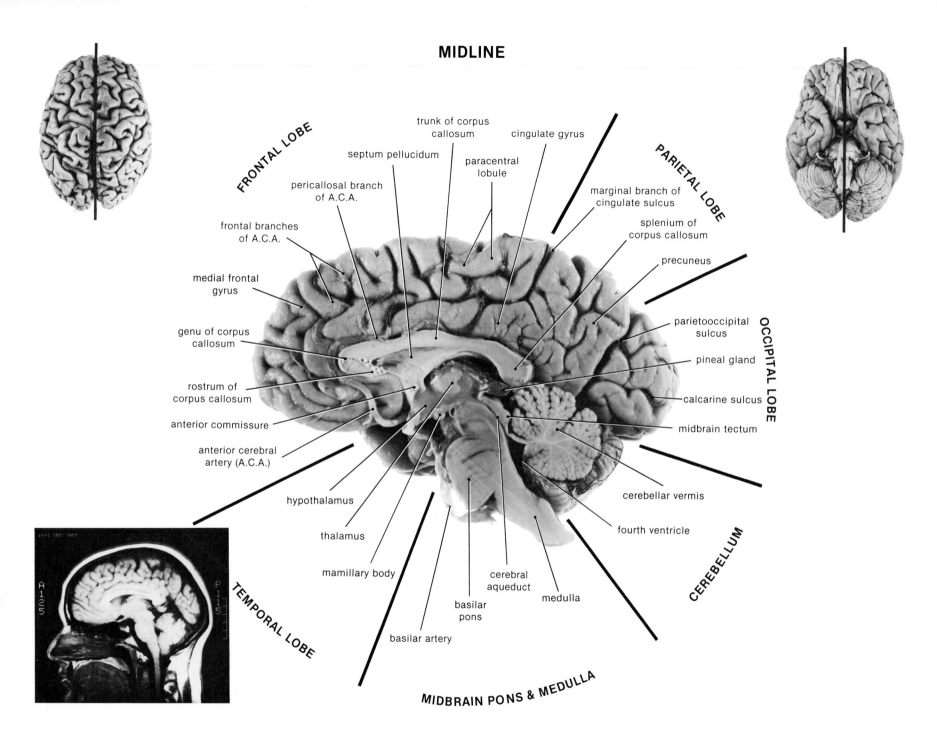

FRONTAL LOBE

trunk of corpus callosum

cingulate gyrus

septum pellucidum

paracentral lobule

PARIETAL LOBE

pericallosal branch of A.C.A.

marginal branch of cingulate sulcus

frontal branches of A.C.A.

splenium of corpus callosum

precuneus

medial frontal gyrus

parietooccipital sulcus

OCCIPITAL LOBE

genu of corpus callosum

pineal gland

rostrum of corpus callosum

calcarine sulcus

anterior commissure

midbrain tectum

anterior cerebral artery (A.C.A.)

cerebellar vermis

hypothalamus

fourth ventricle

thalamus

CEREBELLUM

mamillary body

cerebral aqueduct

medulla

basilar pons

TEMPORAL LOBE

basilar artery

MIDBRAIN PONS & MEDULLA

118

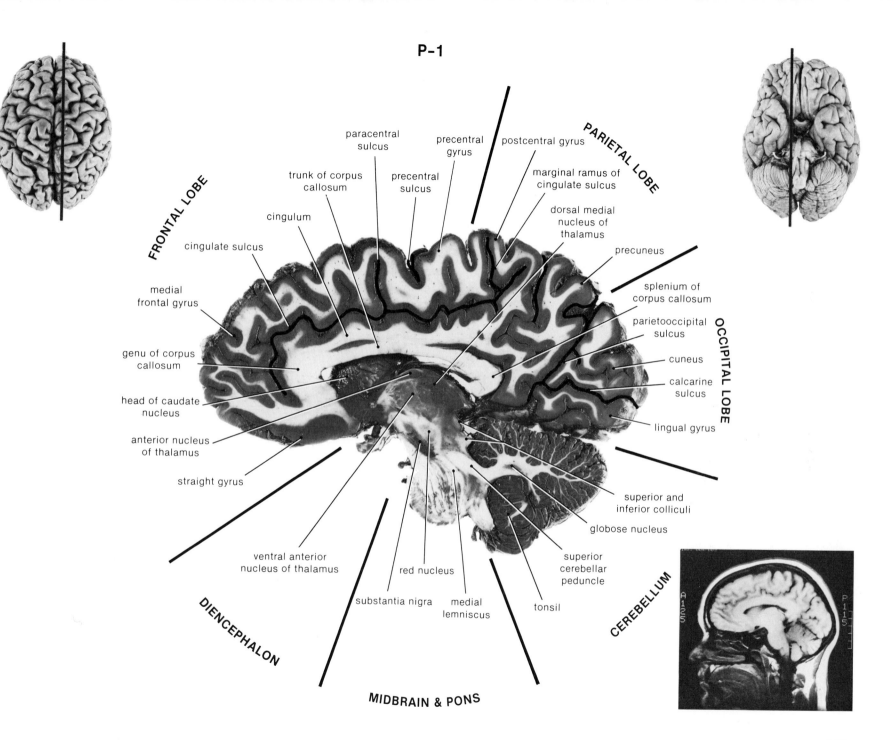

FRONTAL LOBE

PARIETAL LOBE

OCCIPITAL LOBE

CEREBELLUM

DIENCEPHALON

MIDBRAIN & PONS

paracentral sulcus

precentral gyrus

postcentral gyrus

trunk of corpus callosum

precentral sulcus

marginal ramus of cingulate sulcus

cingulum

dorsal medial nucleus of thalamus

cingulate sulcus

precuneus

medial frontal gyrus

splenium of corpus callosum

parietooccipital sulcus

genu of corpus callosum

cuneus

head of caudate nucleus

calcarine sulcus

anterior nucleus of thalamus

lingual gyrus

straight gyrus

superior and inferior colliculi

globose nucleus

superior cerebellar peduncle

ventral anterior nucleus of thalamus

red nucleus

tonsil

substantia nigra

medial lemniscus

119

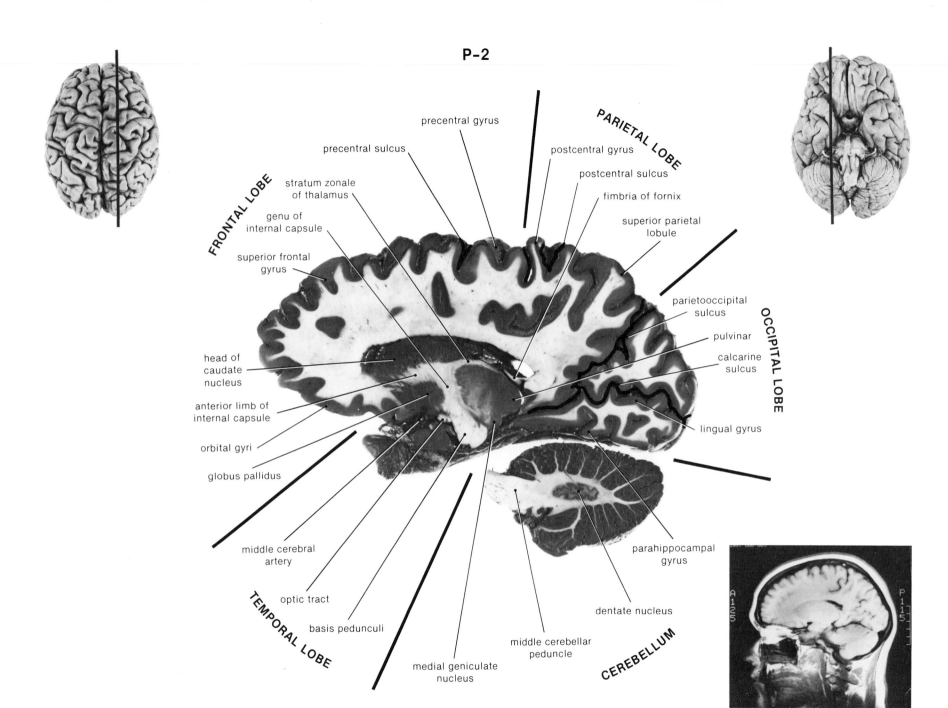

precentral gyrus

PARIETAL LOBE

precentral sulcus

postcentral gyrus

postcentral sulcus

FRONTAL LOBE

stratum zonale of thalamus

fimbria of fornix

genu of internal capsule

superior parietal lobule

superior frontal gyrus

parietooccipital sulcus

OCCIPITAL LOBE

pulvinar

head of caudate nucleus

calcarine sulcus

anterior limb of internal capsule

lingual gyrus

orbital gyri

globus pallidus

middle cerebral artery

parahippocampal gyrus

optic tract

dentate nucleus

TEMPORAL LOBE

basis pedunculi

middle cerebellar peduncle

CEREBELLUM

medial geniculate nucleus

120

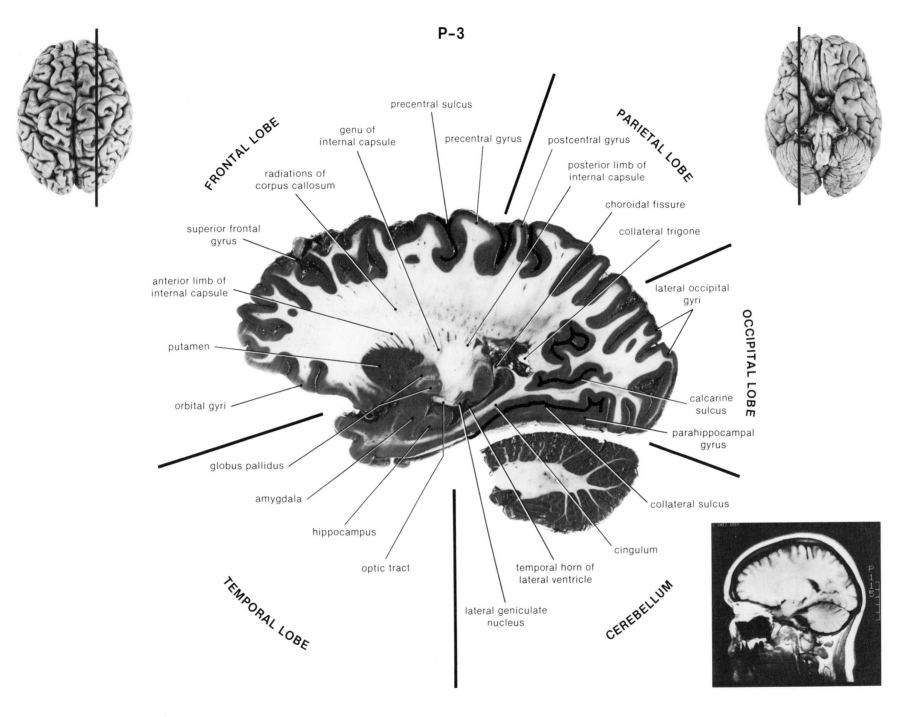

P-3

FRONTAL LOBE

PARIETAL LOBE

OCCIPITAL LOBE

TEMPORAL LOBE

CEREBELLUM

precentral sulcus

genu of internal capsule

precentral gyrus

postcentral gyrus

posterior limb of internal capsule

choroidal fissure

collateral trigone

radiations of corpus callosum

superior frontal gyrus

lateral occipital gyri

anterior limb of internal capsule

putamen

calcarine sulcus

orbital gyri

parahippocampal gyrus

globus pallidus

collateral sulcus

amygdala

hippocampus

cingulum

optic tract

temporal horn of lateral ventricle

lateral geniculate nucleus

P-4

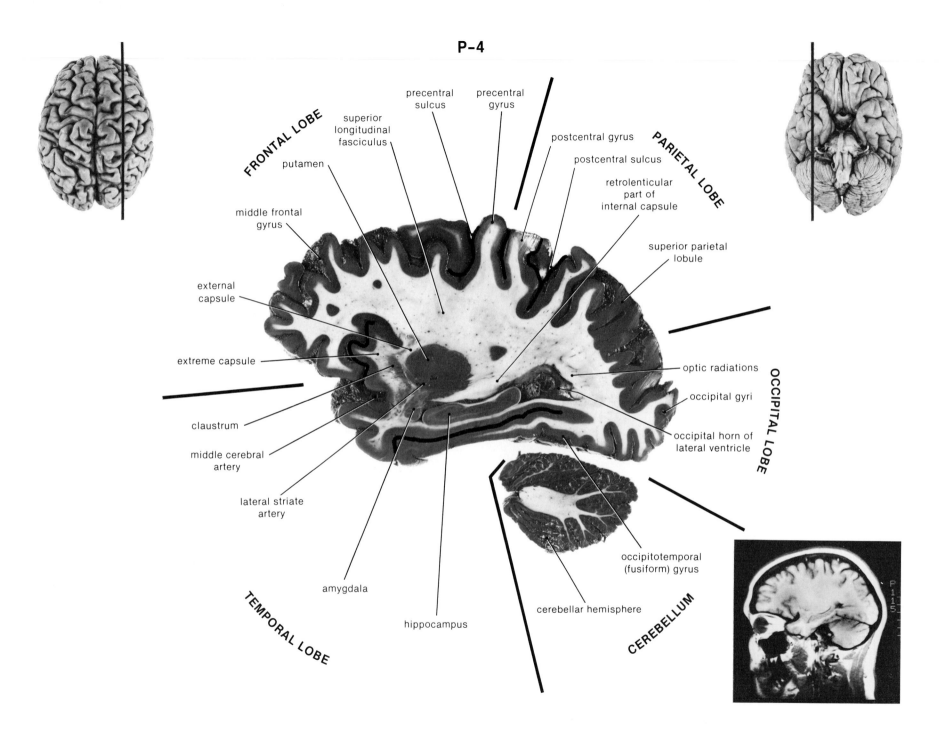

FRONTAL LOBE

PARIETAL LOBE

OCCIPITAL LOBE

CEREBELLUM

TEMPORAL LOBE

precentral sulcus

precentral gyrus

superior longitudinal fasciculus

postcentral gyrus

postcentral sulcus

putamen

retrolenticular part of internal capsule

middle frontal gyrus

superior parietal lobule

external capsule

extreme capsule

optic radiations

occipital gyri

claustrum

occipital horn of lateral ventricle

middle cerebral artery

lateral striate artery

amygdala

occipitotemporal (fusiform) gyrus

hippocampus

cerebellar hemisphere

122

P-5

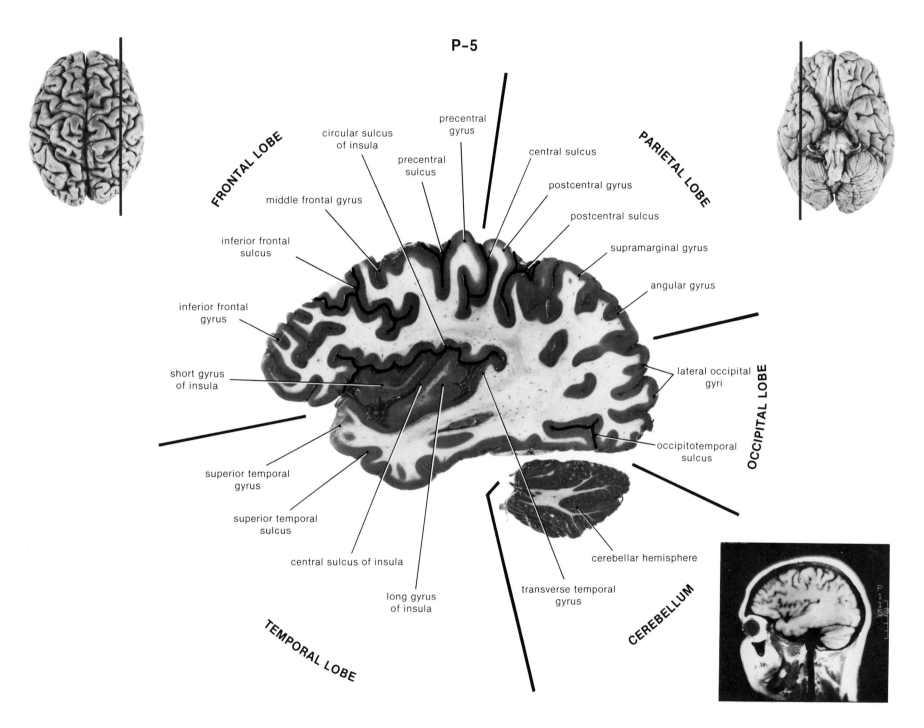

FRONTAL LOBE

PARIETAL LOBE

circular sulcus of insula

precentral gyrus

precentral sulcus

central sulcus

middle frontal gyrus

postcentral gyrus

postcentral sulcus

inferior frontal sulcus

supramarginal gyrus

angular gyrus

inferior frontal gyrus

short gyrus of insula

lateral occipital gyri

occipitotemporal sulcus

OCCIPITAL LOBE

superior temporal gyrus

superior temporal sulcus

central sulcus of insula

long gyrus of insula

transverse temporal gyrus

cerebellar hemisphere

CEREBELLUM

TEMPORAL LOBE

123

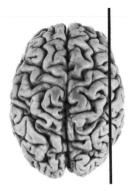

P-6

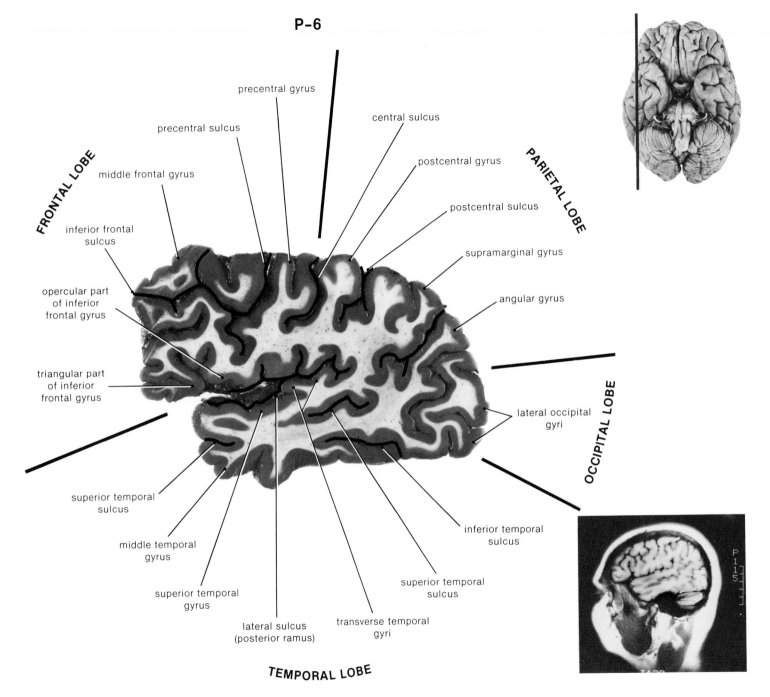

FRONTAL LOBE

PARIETAL LOBE

OCCIPITAL LOBE

TEMPORAL LOBE

precentral gyrus

central sulcus

precentral sulcus

postcentral gyrus

middle frontal gyrus

postcentral sulcus

inferior frontal sulcus

supramarginal gyrus

opercular part of inferior frontal gyrus

angular gyrus

triangular part of inferior frontal gyrus

lateral occipital gyri

superior temporal sulcus

inferior temporal sulcus

middle temporal gyrus

superior temporal sulcus

superior temporal gyrus

lateral sulcus (posterior ramus)

transverse temporal gyri

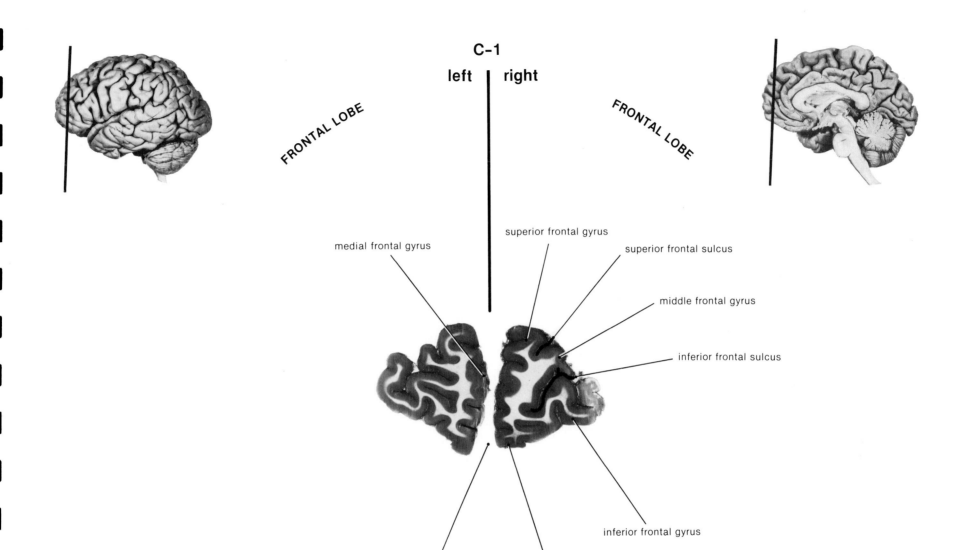

C-1

left | right

FRONTAL LOBE

FRONTAL LOBE

superior frontal gyrus

superior frontal sulcus

medial frontal gyrus

middle frontal gyrus

inferior frontal sulcus

inferior frontal gyrus

straight gyrus

longitudinal cerebral fissure

125

left **right**

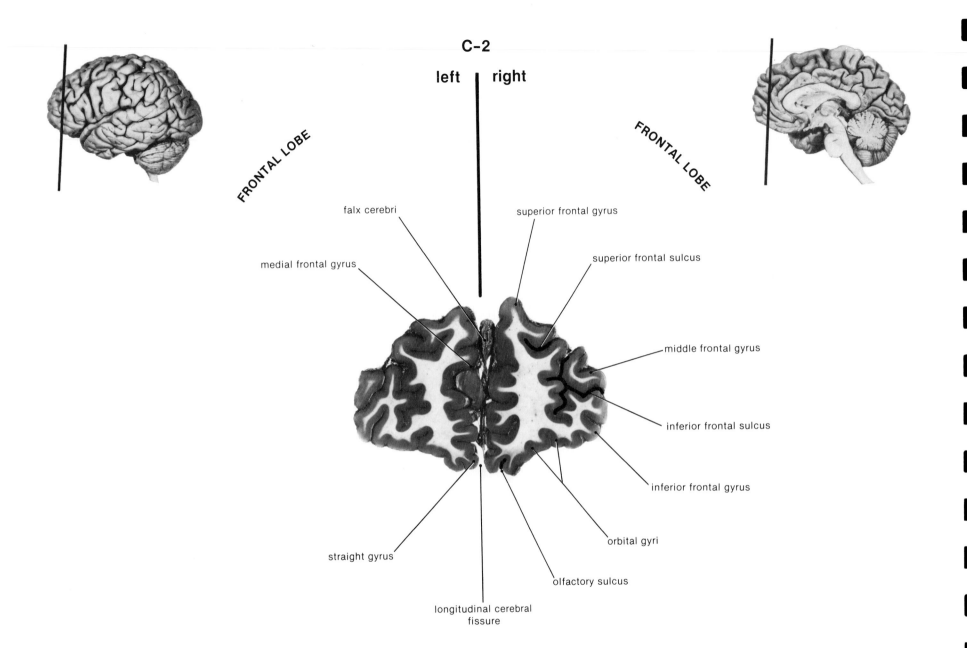

FRONTAL LOBE

FRONTAL LOBE

falx cerebri

superior frontal gyrus

superior frontal sulcus

medial frontal gyrus

middle frontal gyrus

inferior frontal sulcus

inferior frontal gyrus

orbital gyri

straight gyrus

olfactory sulcus

longitudinal cerebral fissure

126

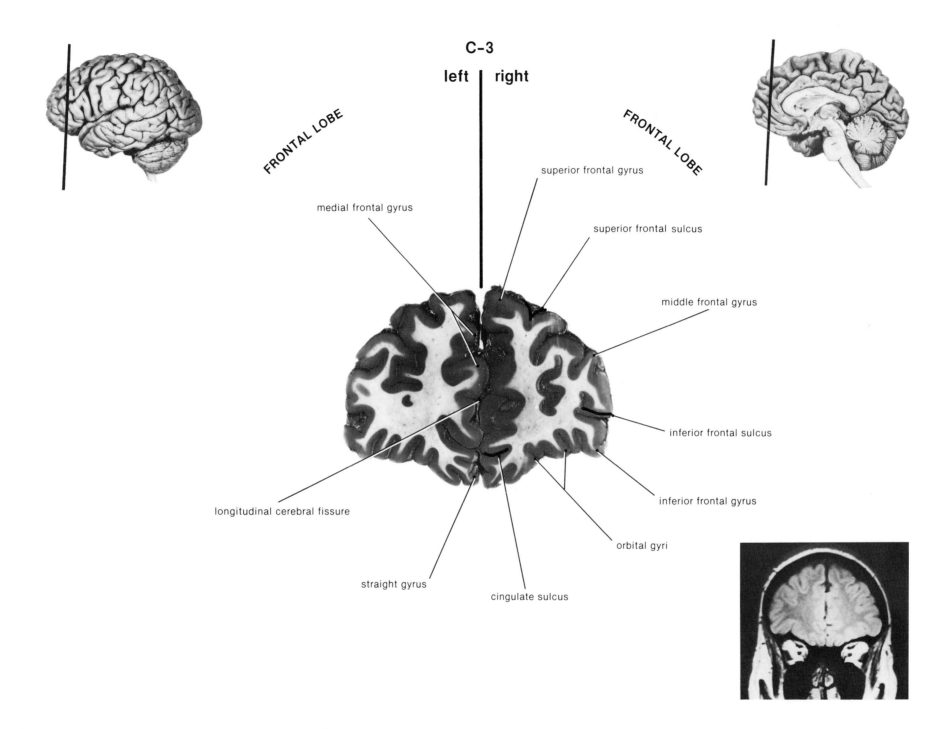

C-3

left | right

FRONTAL LOBE

FRONTAL LOBE

superior frontal gyrus

medial frontal gyrus

superior frontal sulcus

middle frontal gyrus

inferior frontal sulcus

longitudinal cerebral fissure

inferior frontal gyrus

orbital gyri

straight gyrus

cingulate sulcus

127

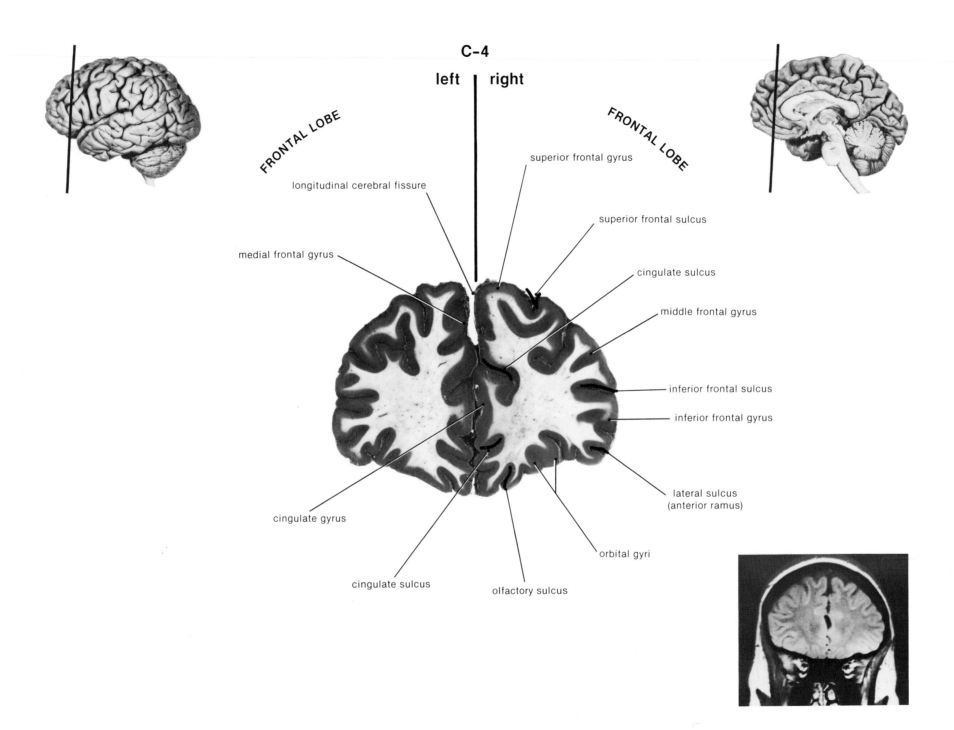

C-4

left | right

FRONTAL LOBE

FRONTAL LOBE

longitudinal cerebral fissure

superior frontal gyrus

superior frontal sulcus

medial frontal gyrus

cingulate sulcus

middle frontal gyrus

inferior frontal sulcus

inferior frontal gyrus

lateral sulcus
(anterior ramus)

cingulate gyrus

orbital gyri

cingulate sulcus

olfactory sulcus

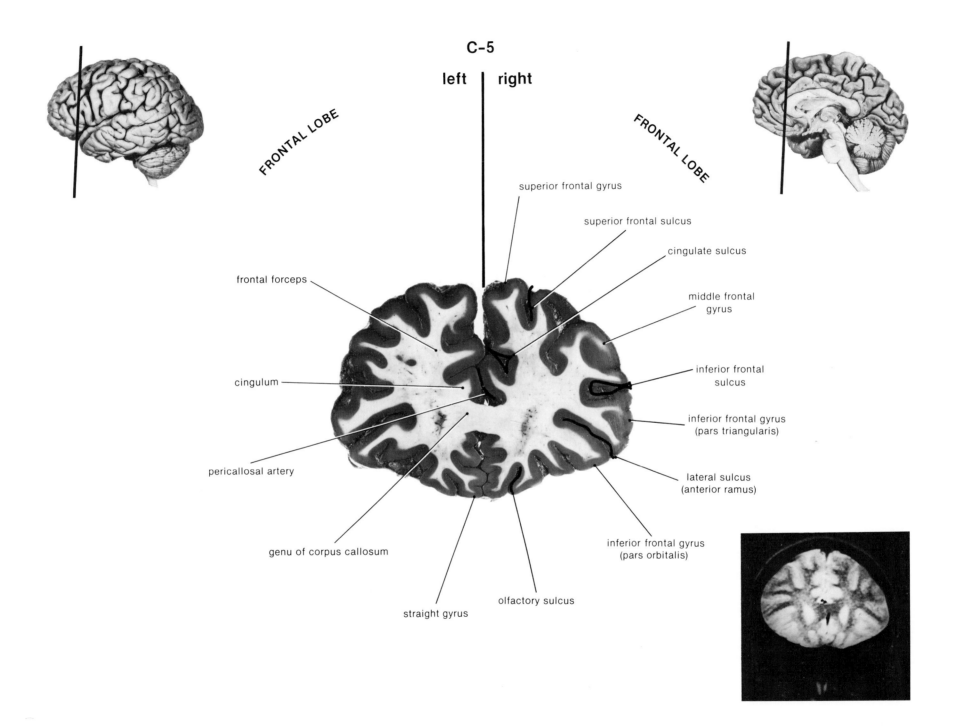

FRONTAL LOBE

FRONTAL LOBE

superior frontal gyrus

superior frontal sulcus

cingulate sulcus

middle frontal gyrus

frontal forceps

inferior frontal sulcus

cingulum

inferior frontal gyrus (pars triangularis)

lateral sulcus (anterior ramus)

pericallosal artery

inferior frontal gyrus (pars orbitalis)

genu of corpus callosum

olfactory sulcus

straight gyrus

left | right

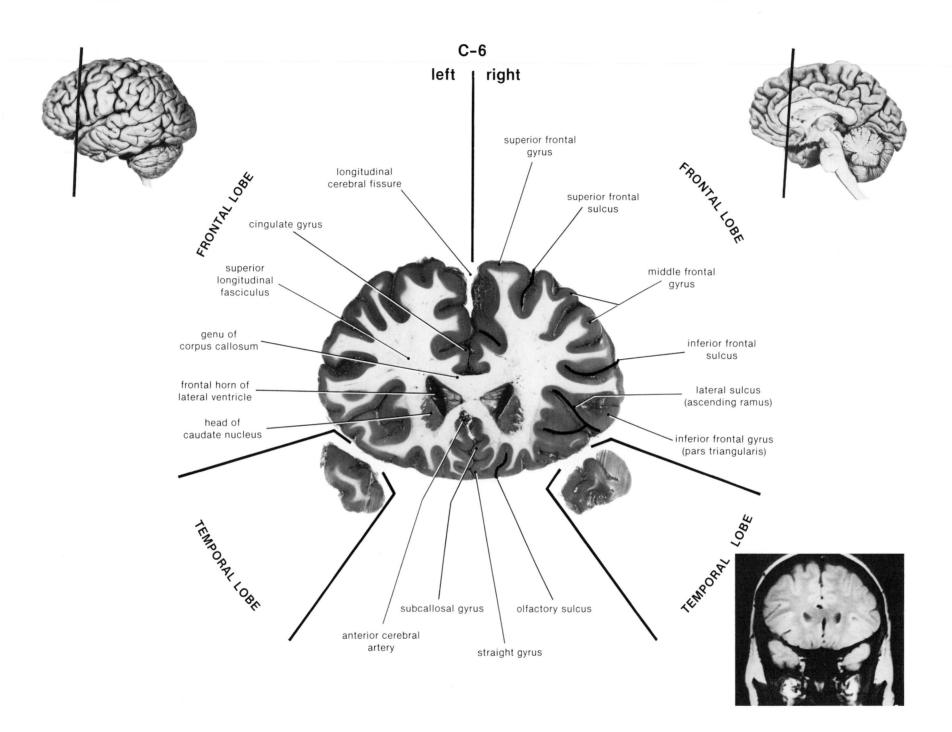

FRONTAL LOBE

longitudinal
cerebral fissure

superior frontal
gyrus

superior frontal
sulcus

cingulate gyrus

FRONTAL LOBE

middle frontal
gyrus

superior
longitudinal
fasciculus

inferior frontal
sulcus

genu of
corpus callosum

lateral sulcus
(ascending ramus)

frontal horn of
lateral ventricle

head of
caudate nucleus

inferior frontal gyrus
(pars triangularis)

TEMPORAL LOBE

TEMPORAL LOBE

subcallosal gyrus

olfactory sulcus

anterior cerebral
artery

straight gyrus

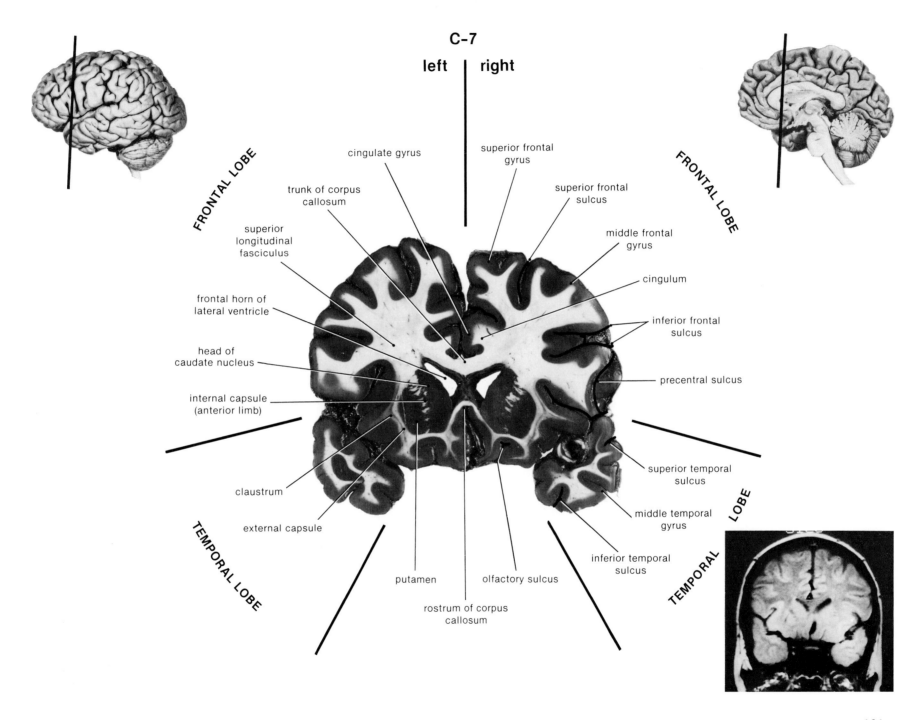

C-7

left | right

FRONTAL LOBE

cingulate gyrus

superior frontal gyrus

trunk of corpus callosum

superior frontal sulcus

superior longitudinal fasciculus

middle frontal gyrus

FRONTAL LOBE

frontal horn of lateral ventricle

cingulum

head of caudate nucleus

inferior frontal sulcus

internal capsule (anterior limb)

precentral sulcus

claustrum

superior temporal sulcus

external capsule

middle temporal gyrus

putamen

inferior temporal sulcus

TEMPORAL LOBE

olfactory sulcus

TEMPORAL LOBE

rostrum of corpus callosum

TEMPORAL LOBE

131

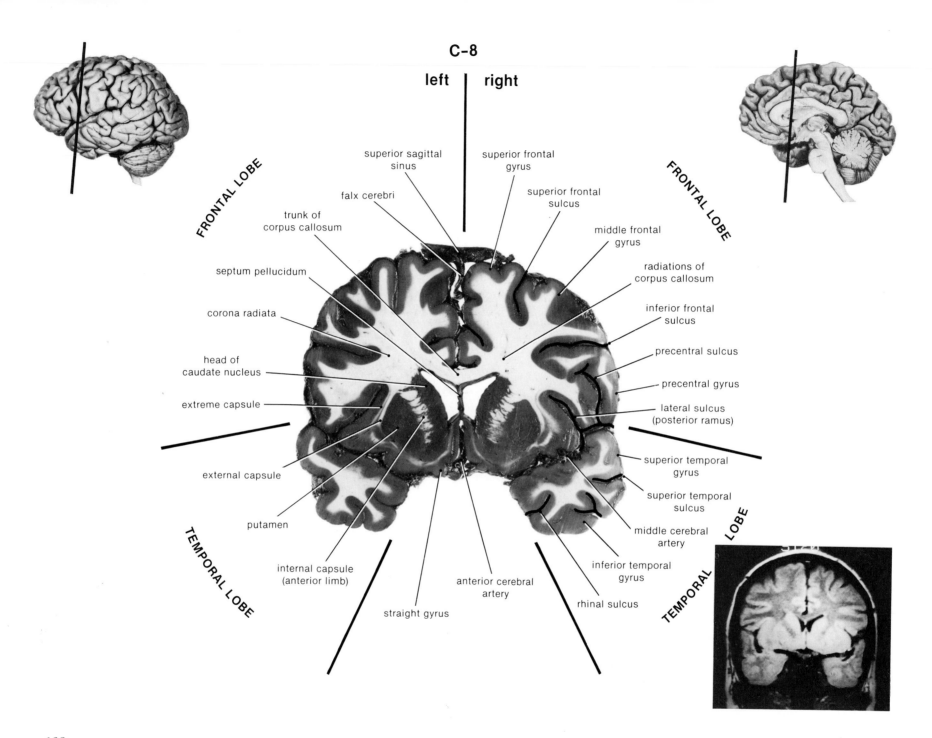

C-8

left | right

FRONTAL LOBE

FRONTAL LOBE

superior sagittal sinus

superior frontal gyrus

superior frontal sulcus

falx cerebri

trunk of corpus callosum

middle frontal gyrus

septum pellucidum

radiations of corpus callosum

corona radiata

inferior frontal sulcus

precentral sulcus

head of caudate nucleus

precentral gyrus

extreme capsule

lateral sulcus (posterior ramus)

external capsule

superior temporal gyrus

putamen

superior temporal sulcus

middle cerebral artery

internal capsule (anterior limb)

anterior cerebral artery

inferior temporal gyrus

straight gyrus

rhinal sulcus

TEMPORAL LOBE

TEMPORAL LOBE

132

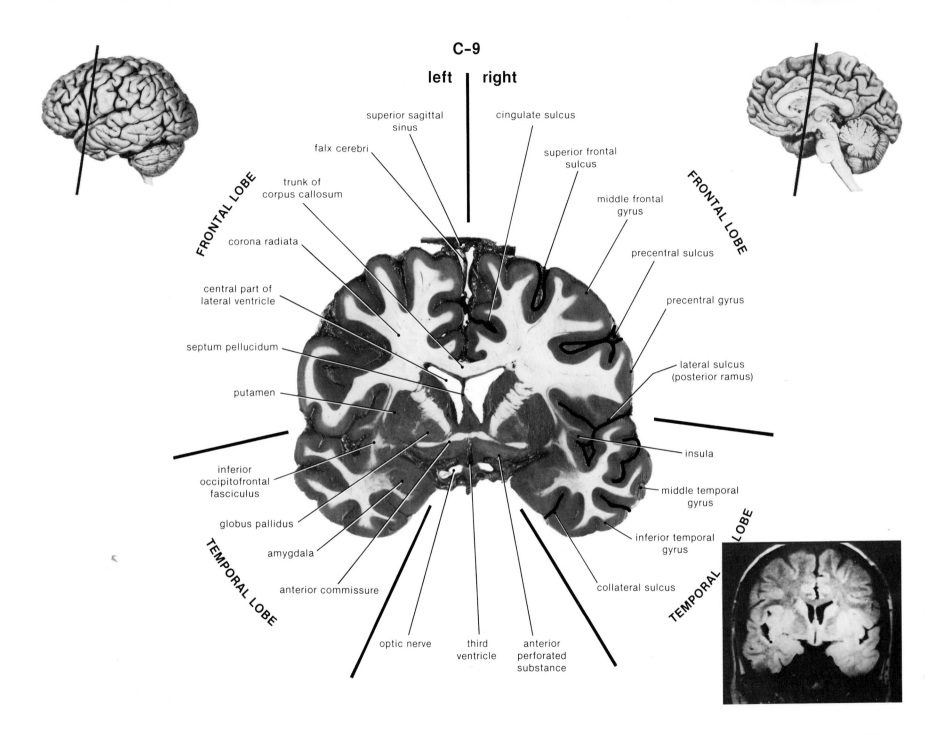

superior sagittal
sinus

cingulate sulcus

falx cerebri

superior frontal
sulcus

FRONTAL LOBE

trunk of
corpus callosum

middle frontal
gyrus

FRONTAL LOBE

corona radiata

precentral sulcus

central part of
lateral ventricle

precentral gyrus

septum pellucidum

lateral sulcus
(posterior ramus)

putamen

insula

inferior
occipitofrontal
fasciculus

middle temporal
gyrus

globus pallidus

inferior temporal
gyrus

TEMPORAL LOBE

amygdala

TEMPORAL LOBE

anterior commissure

collateral sulcus

optic nerve

third
ventricle

anterior
perforated
substance

133

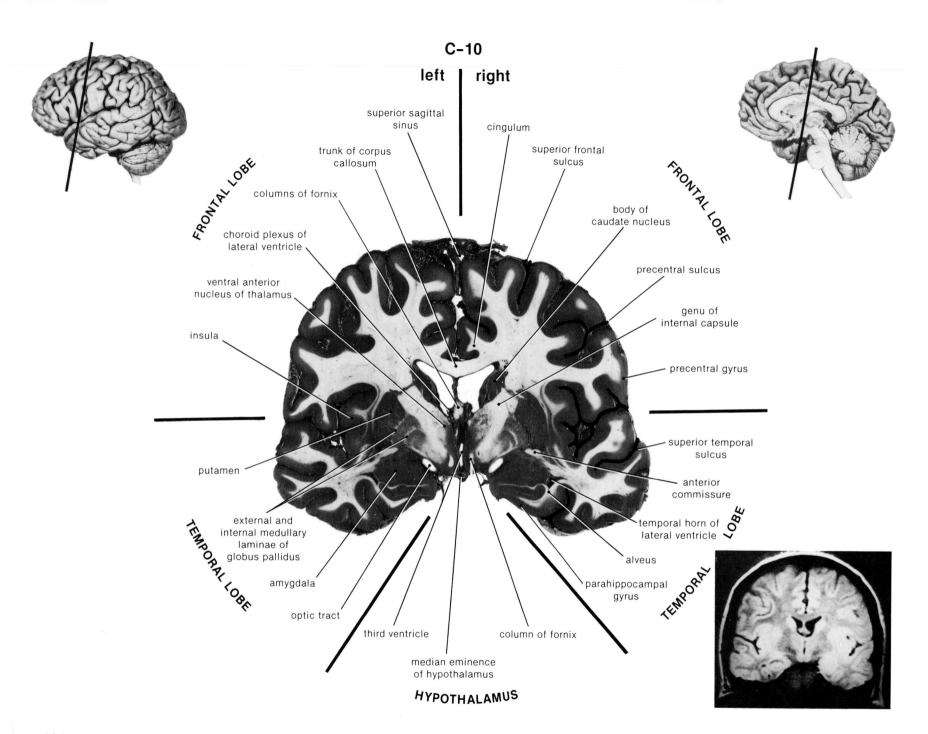

superior sagittal sinus

cingulum

trunk of corpus callosum

superior frontal sulcus

FRONTAL LOBE

FRONTAL LOBE

columns of fornix

body of caudate nucleus

choroid plexus of lateral ventricle

precentral sulcus

ventral anterior nucleus of thalamus

genu of internal capsule

insula

precentral gyrus

putamen

superior temporal sulcus

external and internal medullary laminae of globus pallidus

anterior commissure

temporal horn of lateral ventricle

amygdala

TEMPORAL LOBE

TEMPORAL LOBE

alveus

optic tract

parahippocampal gyrus

third ventricle

column of fornix

median eminence of hypothalamus

HYPOTHALAMUS

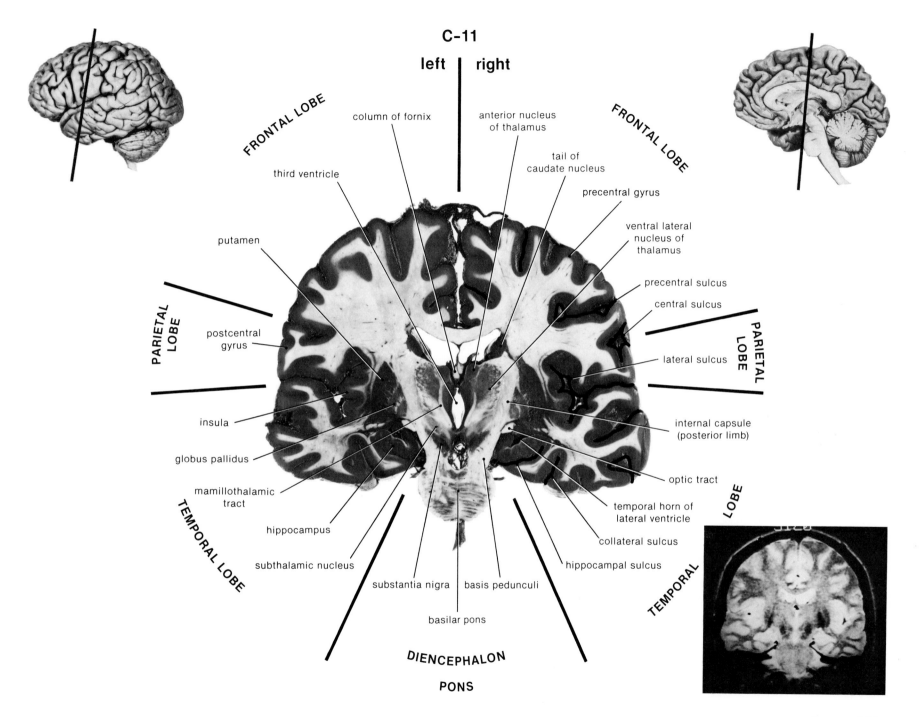

left | **right**

FRONTAL LOBE

column of fornix

anterior nucleus of thalamus

FRONTAL LOBE

third ventricle

tail of caudate nucleus

precentral gyrus

putamen

ventral lateral nucleus of thalamus

PARIETAL LOBE

precentral sulcus

central sulcus

postcentral gyrus

PARIETAL LOBE

lateral sulcus

insula

internal capsule (posterior limb)

globus pallidus

optic tract

mamillothalamic tract

temporal horn of lateral ventricle

TEMPORAL LOBE

hippocampus

collateral sulcus

subthalamic nucleus

hippocampal sulcus

TEMPORAL LOBE

substantia nigra

basis pedunculi

basilar pons

DIENCEPHALON

PONS

135

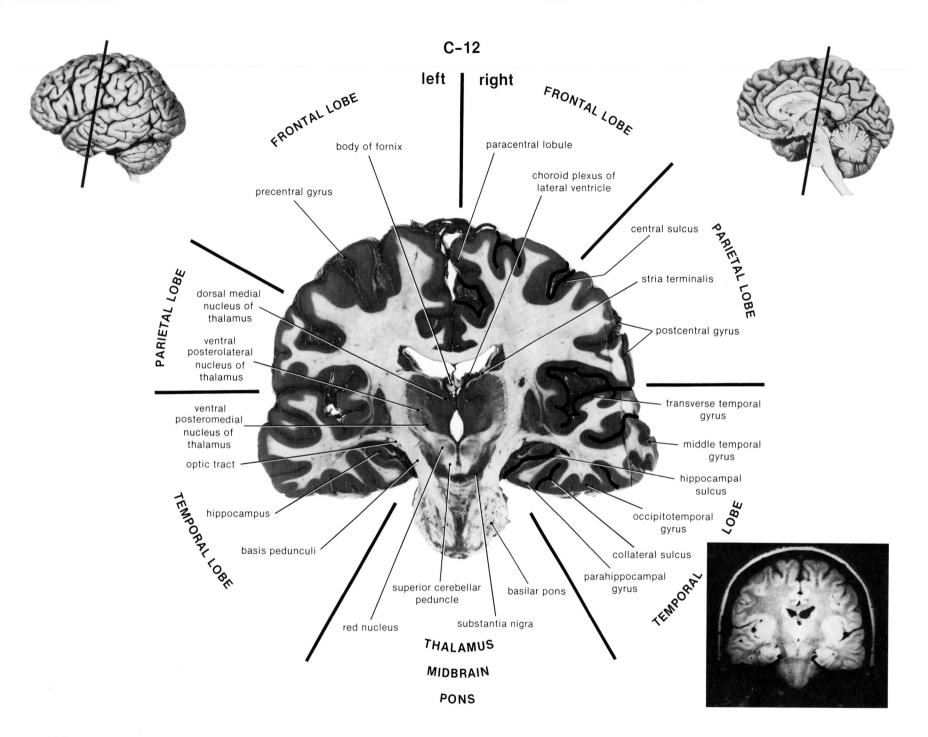

left right

FRONTAL LOBE

FRONTAL LOBE

body of fornix

paracentral lobule

precentral gyrus

choroid plexus of lateral ventricle

central sulcus

PARIETAL LOBE

stria terminalis

PARIETAL LOBE

dorsal medial nucleus of thalamus

postcentral gyrus

ventral posterolateral nucleus of thalamus

transverse temporal gyrus

ventral posteromedial nucleus of thalamus

postcentral gyrus

optic tract

middle temporal gyrus

hippocampal sulcus

TEMPORAL LOBE

hippocampus

occipitotemporal gyrus

basis pedunculi

collateral sulcus

TEMPORAL LOBE

parahippocampal gyrus

superior cerebellar peduncle

basilar pons

TEMPORAL

red nucleus

substantia nigra

THALAMUS

MIDBRAIN

PONS

136

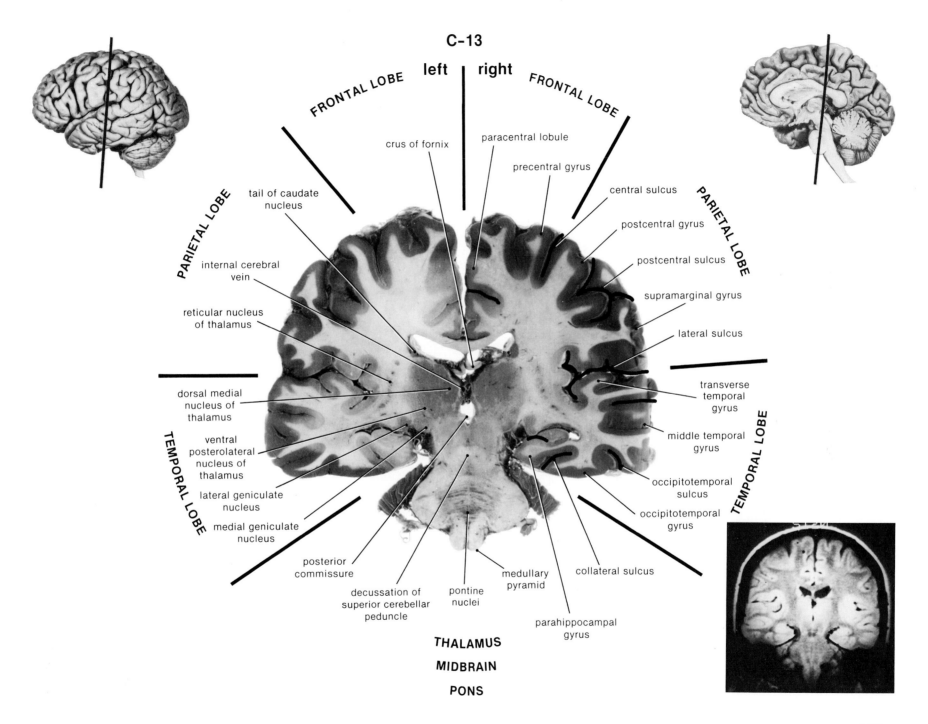

left   right

FRONTAL LOBE

FRONTAL LOBE

FRONTAL LOBE

PARIETAL LOBE

PARIETAL LOBE

PARIETAL LOBE

TEMPORAL LOBE

TEMPORAL LOBE

crus of fornix

paracentral lobule

precentral gyrus

central sulcus

postcentral gyrus

postcentral sulcus

supramarginal gyrus

lateral sulcus

tail of caudate nucleus

internal cerebral vein

reticular nucleus of thalamus

dorsal medial nucleus of thalamus

ventral posterolateral nucleus of thalamus

lateral geniculate nucleus

medial geniculate nucleus

transverse temporal gyrus

middle temporal gyrus

occipitotemporal sulcus

occipitotemporal gyrus

posterior commissure

decussation of superior cerebellar peduncle

pontine nuclei

medullary pyramid

collateral sulcus

parahippocampal gyrus

THALAMUS

MIDBRAIN

PONS

137

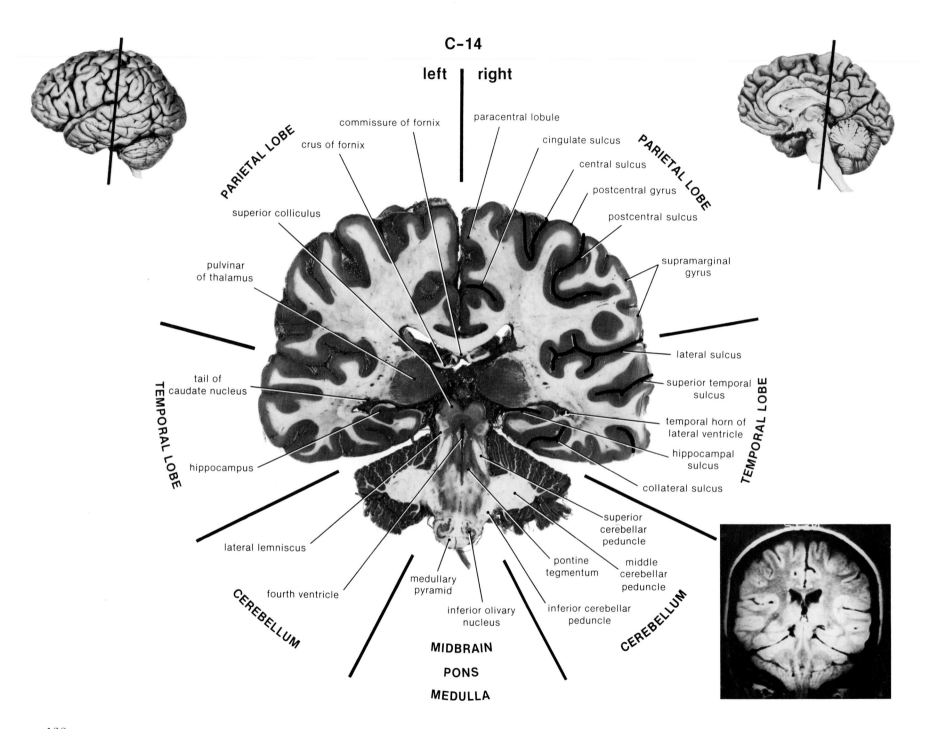

left | right

PARIETAL LOBE

commissure of fornix

crus of fornix

paracentral lobule

cingulate sulcus

central sulcus

postcentral gyrus

postcentral sulcus

PARIETAL LOBE

superior colliculus

supramarginal gyrus

pulvinar of thalamus

lateral sulcus

superior temporal sulcus

TEMPORAL LOBE

tail of caudate nucleus

temporal horn of lateral ventricle

hippocampal sulcus

TEMPORAL LOBE

collateral sulcus

hippocampus

superior cerebellar peduncle

lateral lemniscus

CEREBELLUM

fourth ventricle

medullary pyramid

inferior olivary nucleus

pontine tegmentum

middle cerebellar peduncle

inferior cerebellar peduncle

CEREBELLUM

MIDBRAIN

PONS

MEDULLA

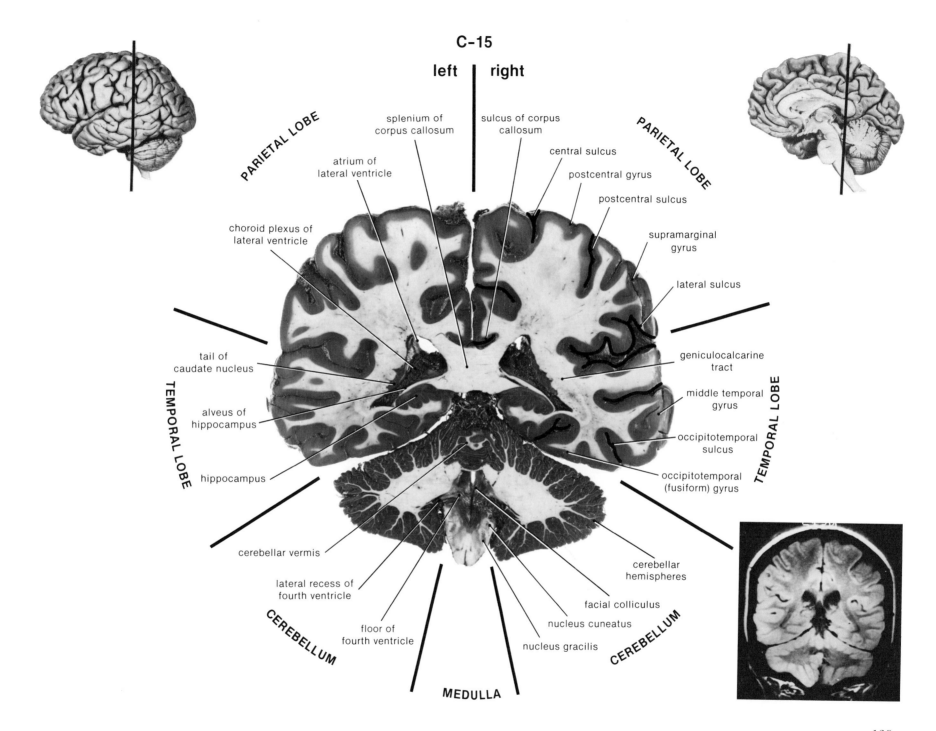

C-15

left   right

PARIETAL LOBE

PARIETAL LOBE

TEMPORAL LOBE

TEMPORAL LOBE

CEREBELLUM

CEREBELLUM

MEDULLA

splenium of corpus callosum

atrium of lateral ventricle

choroid plexus of lateral ventricle

tail of caudate nucleus

alveus of hippocampus

hippocampus

cerebellar vermis

lateral recess of fourth ventricle

floor of fourth ventricle

sulcus of corpus callosum

central sulcus

postcentral gyrus

postcentral sulcus

supramarginal gyrus

lateral sulcus

geniculocalcarine tract

middle temporal gyrus

occipitotemporal sulcus

occipitotemporal (fusiform) gyrus

cerebellar hemispheres

facial colliculus

nucleus cuneatus

nucleus gracilis

139

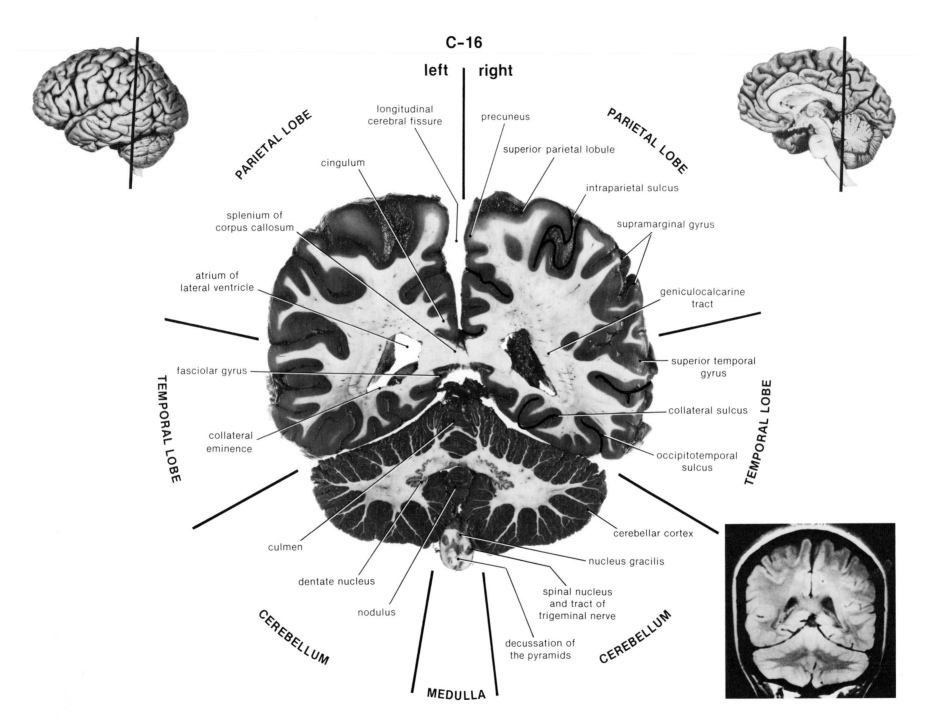

C-16

left right

longitudinal cerebral fissure · precuneus

PARIETAL LOBE · PARIETAL LOBE

cingulum · superior parietal lobule

intraparietal sulcus

splenium of corpus callosum · supramarginal gyrus

atrium of lateral ventricle · geniculocalcarine tract

superior temporal gyrus

fasciolar gyrus

collateral sulcus

TEMPORAL LOBE · TEMPORAL LOBE

collateral eminence · occipitotemporal sulcus

cerebellar cortex

culmen · nucleus gracilis

dentate nucleus · spinal nucleus and tract of trigeminal nerve

CEREBELLUM · CEREBELLUM

nodulus · decussation of the pyramids

MEDULLA

140

left **right**

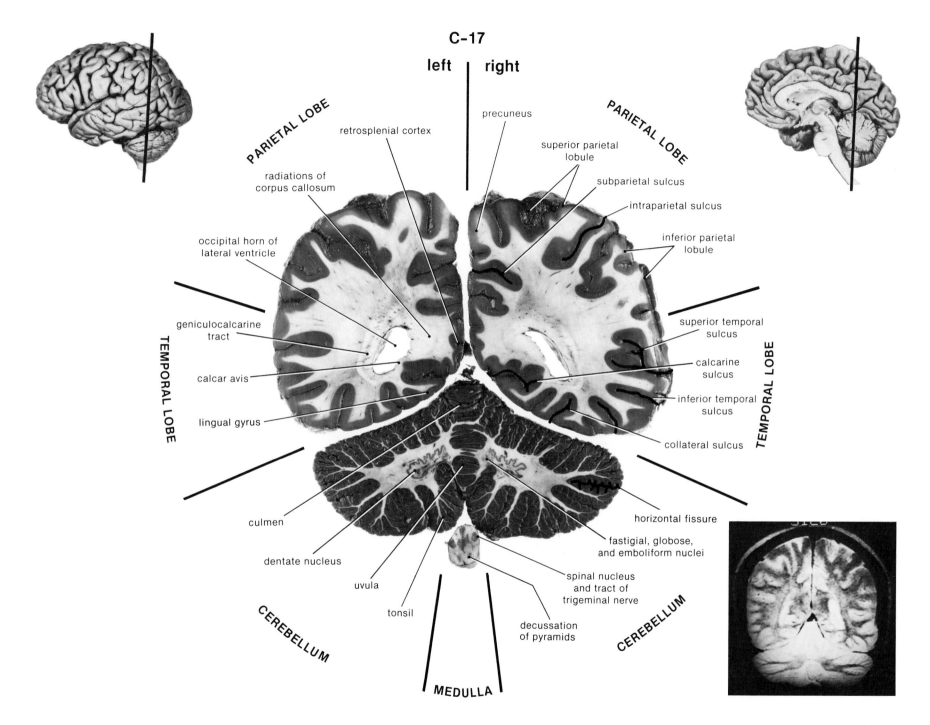

PARIETAL LOBE

retrosplenial cortex

precuneus

PARIETAL LOBE

superior parietal lobule

subparietal sulcus

radiations of corpus callosum

intraparietal sulcus

occipital horn of lateral ventricle

inferior parietal lobule

TEMPORAL LOBE

geniculocalcarine tract

superior temporal sulcus

calcar avis

calcarine sulcus

lingual gyrus

inferior temporal sulcus

collateral sulcus

TEMPORAL LOBE

horizontal fissure

culmen

fastigial, globose, and emboliform nuclei

dentate nucleus

spinal nucleus and tract of trigeminal nerve

uvula

tonsil

decussation of pyramids

CEREBELLUM

CEREBELLUM

MEDULLA

141

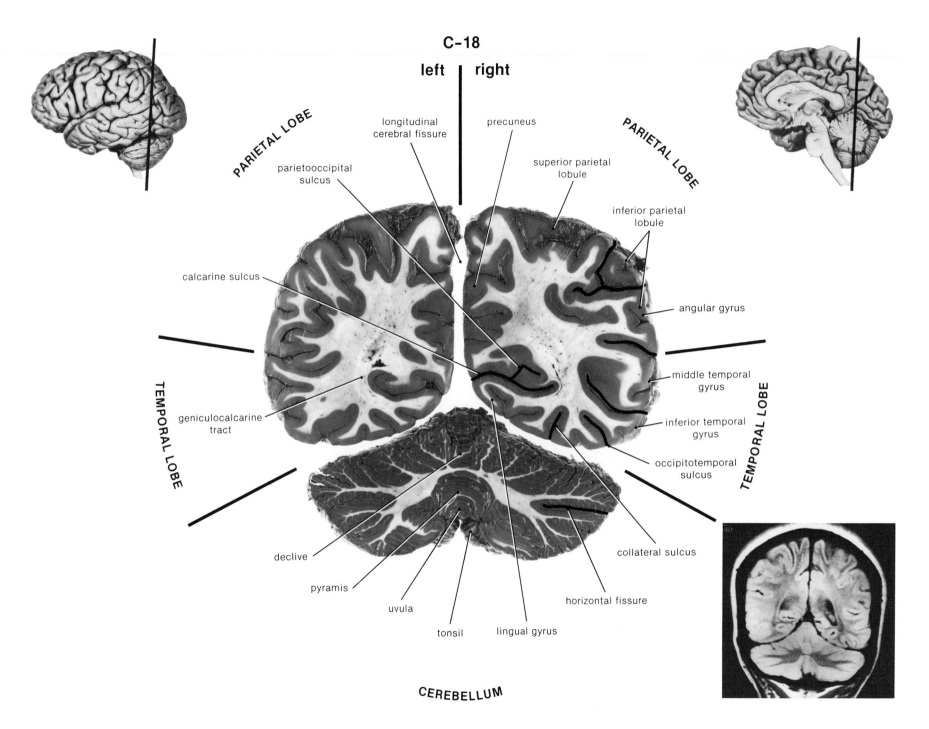

C-18

left | right

PARIETAL LOBE

PARIETAL LOBE

longitudinal cerebral fissure

precuneus

parietooccipital sulcus

superior parietal lobule

inferior parietal lobule

calcarine sulcus

angular gyrus

TEMPORAL LOBE

middle temporal gyrus

geniculocalcarine tract

inferior temporal gyrus

occipitotemporal sulcus

TEMPORAL LOBE

collateral sulcus

declive

horizontal fissure

pyramis

uvula

tonsil

lingual gyrus

CEREBELLUM

142

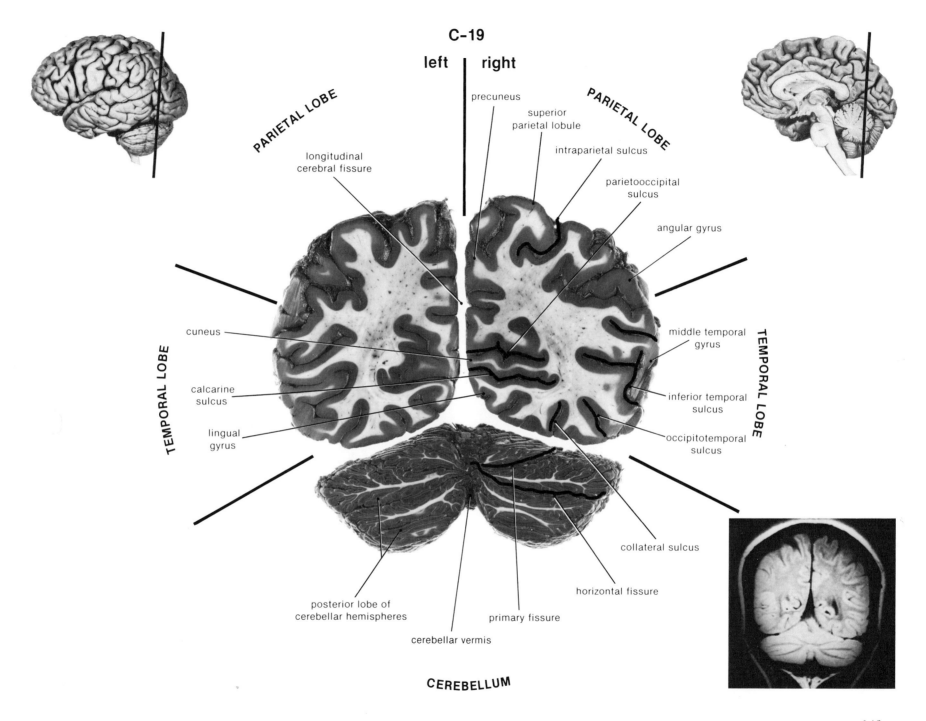

left   **right**

PARIETAL LOBE

PARIETAL LOBE

precuneus

superior
parietal lobule

intraparietal sulcus

parietooccipital
sulcus

longitudinal
cerebral fissure

angular gyrus

cuneus

middle temporal
gyrus

TEMPORAL LOBE

TEMPORAL LOBE

calcarine
sulcus

inferior temporal
sulcus

lingual
gyrus

occipitotemporal
sulcus

collateral sulcus

horizontal fissure

posterior lobe of
cerebellar hemispheres

primary fissure

cerebellar vermis

CEREBELLUM

143

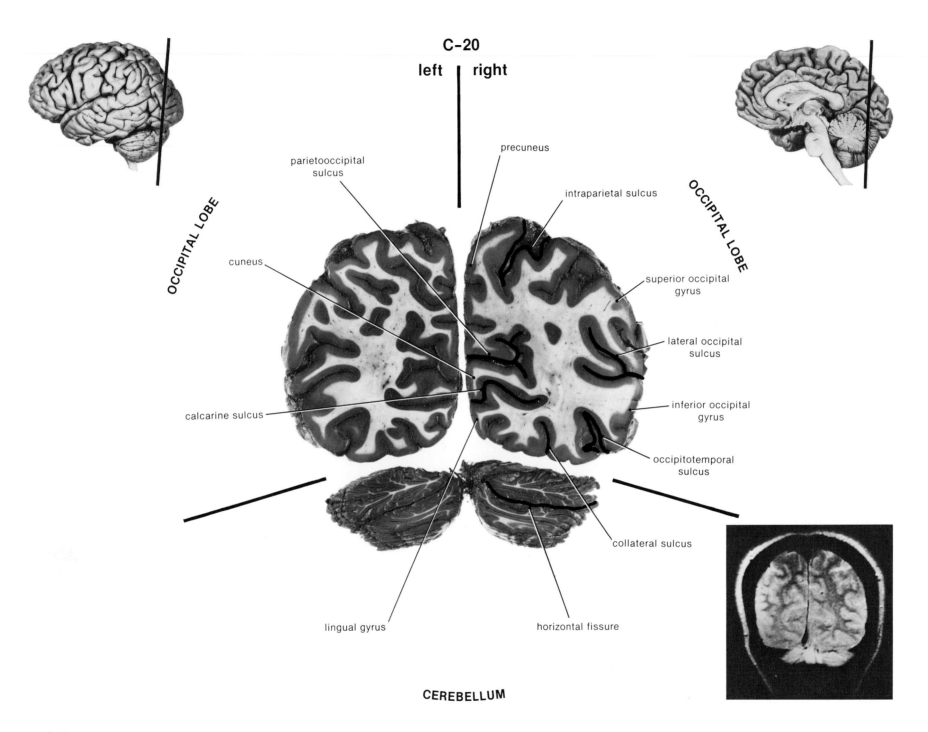

OCCIPITAL LOBE

OCCIPITAL LOBE

precuneus

parietooccipital sulcus

intraparietal sulcus

cuneus

superior occipital gyrus

lateral occipital sulcus

calcarine sulcus

inferior occipital gyrus

occipitotemporal sulcus

collateral sulcus

lingual gyrus

horizontal fissure

CEREBELLUM

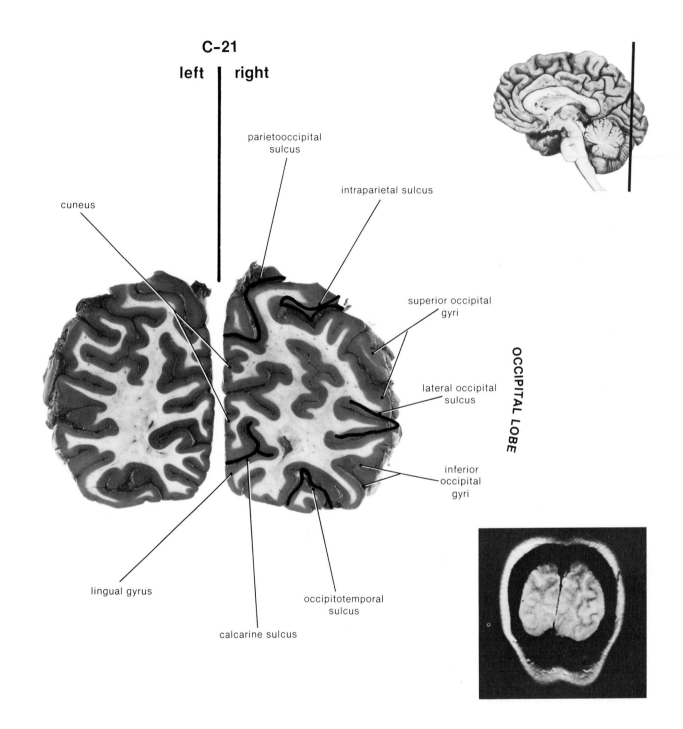

C-21

left | **right**

parietooccipital sulcus

intraparietal sulcus

cuneus

superior occipital gyri

lateral occipital sulcus

inferior occipital gyri

OCCIPITAL LOBE

OCCIPITAL LOBE

lingual gyrus

occipitotemporal sulcus

calcarine sulcus

145

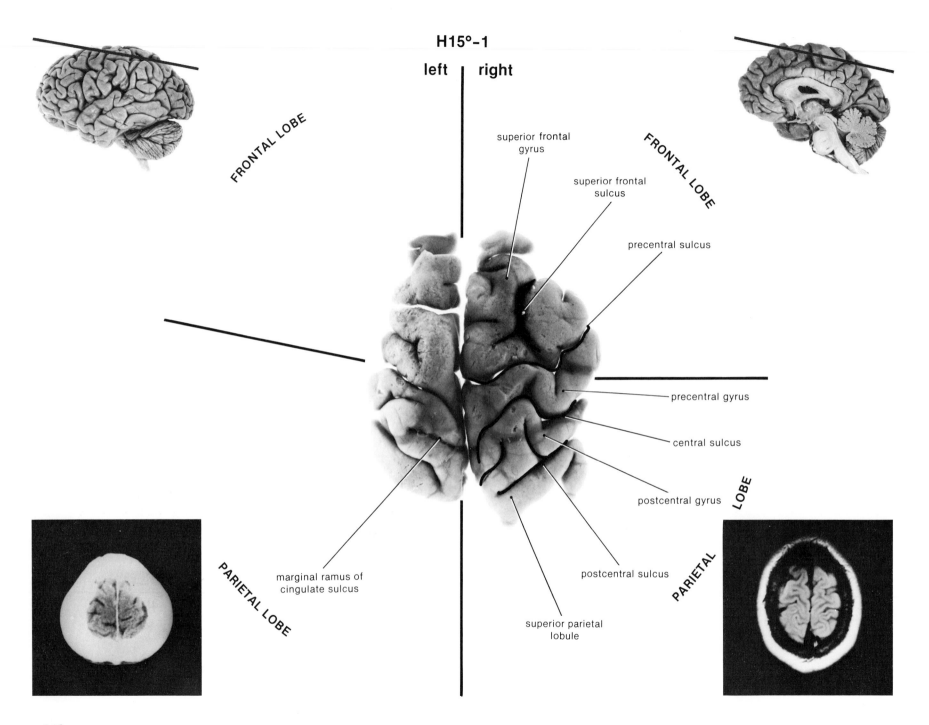

left | right

FRONTAL LOBE

FRONTAL LOBE

superior frontal
gyrus

superior frontal
sulcus

precentral sulcus

precentral gyrus

central sulcus

postcentral gyrus

PARIETAL LOBE

marginal ramus of
cingulate sulcus

postcentral sulcus

superior parietal
lobule

PARIETAL LOBE

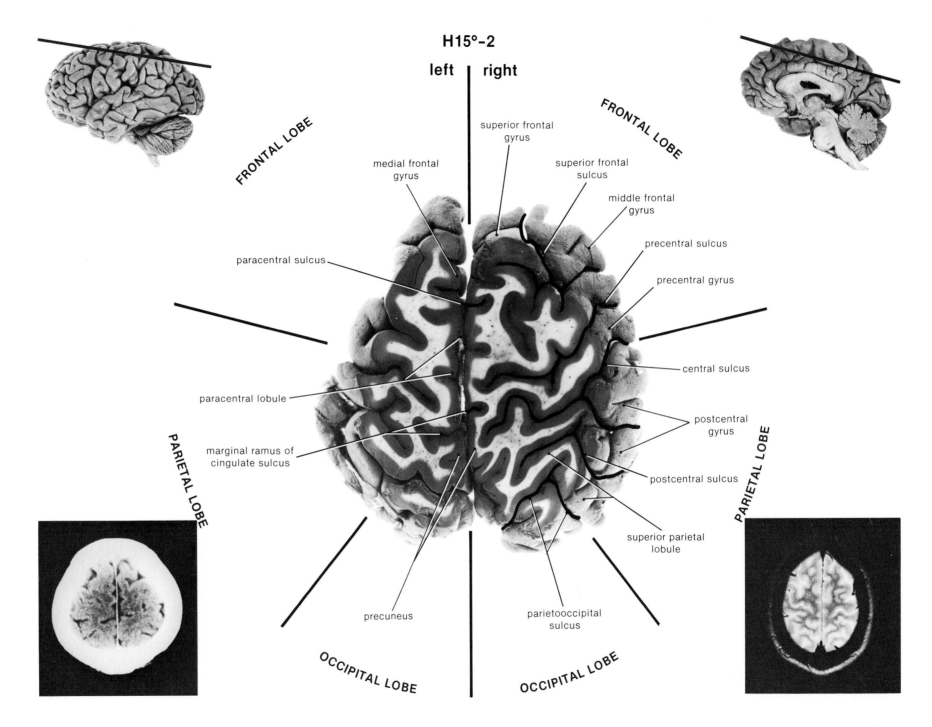

H15°-2

left | right

FRONTAL LOBE

FRONTAL LOBE

superior frontal gyrus

medial frontal gyrus

superior frontal sulcus

middle frontal gyrus

paracentral sulcus

precentral sulcus

precentral gyrus

central sulcus

paracentral lobule

postcentral gyrus

marginal ramus of cingulate sulcus

postcentral sulcus

PARIETAL LOBE

PARIETAL LOBE

superior parietal lobule

precuneus

parietooccipital sulcus

OCCIPITAL LOBE

OCCIPITAL LOBE

147

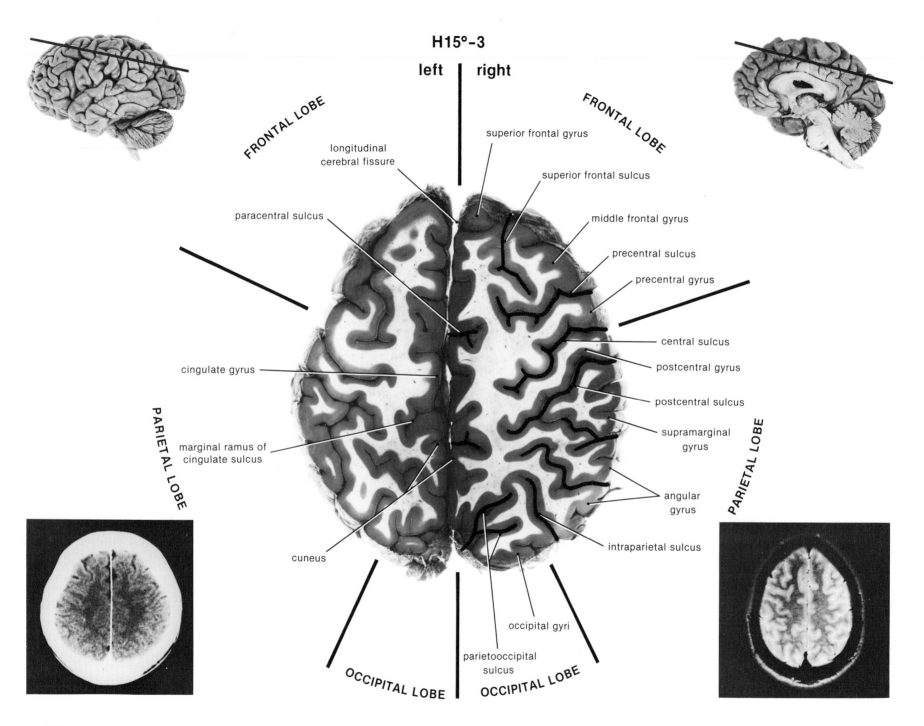

FRONTAL LOBE

FRONTAL LOBE

longitudinal cerebral fissure

superior frontal gyrus

superior frontal sulcus

paracentral sulcus

middle frontal gyrus

precentral sulcus

precentral gyrus

central sulcus

postcentral gyrus

cingulate gyrus

postcentral sulcus

supramarginal gyrus

marginal ramus of cingulate sulcus

angular gyrus

intraparietal sulcus

cuneus

occipital gyri

parietooccipital sulcus

PARIETAL LOBE

PARIETAL LOBE

OCCIPITAL LOBE

OCCIPITAL LOBE

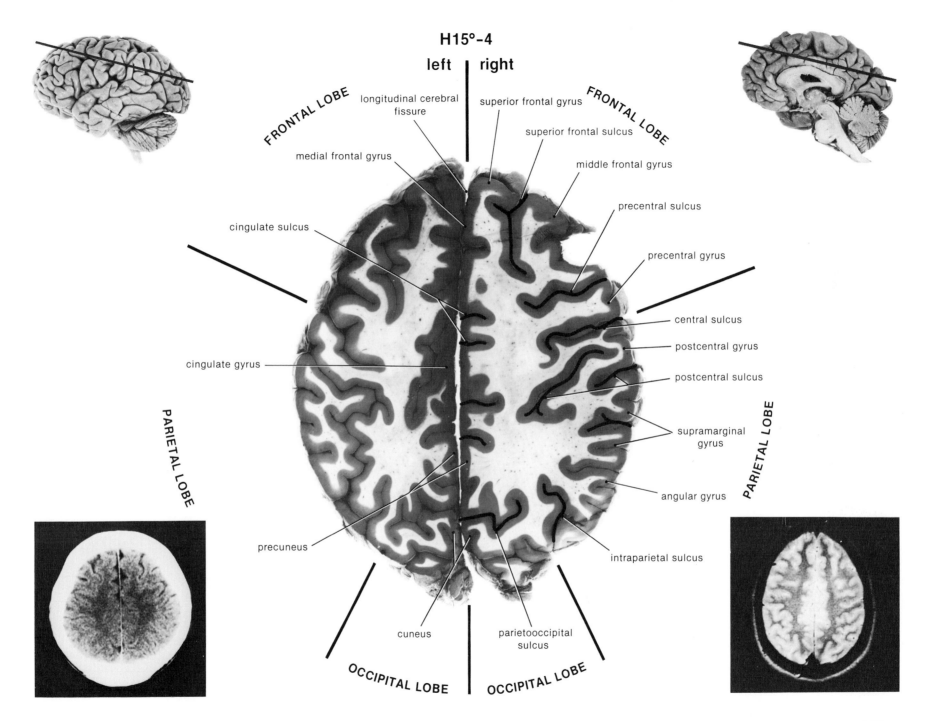

H15°-4

left | right

FRONTAL LOBE

longitudinal cerebral fissure

superior frontal gyrus

FRONTAL LOBE

medial frontal gyrus

superior frontal sulcus

middle frontal gyrus

cingulate sulcus

precentral sulcus

precentral gyrus

central sulcus

postcentral gyrus

cingulate gyrus

postcentral sulcus

supramarginal gyrus

PARIETAL LOBE

PARIETAL LOBE

angular gyrus

precuneus

intraparietal sulcus

cuneus

parietooccipital sulcus

OCCIPITAL LOBE

OCCIPITAL LOBE

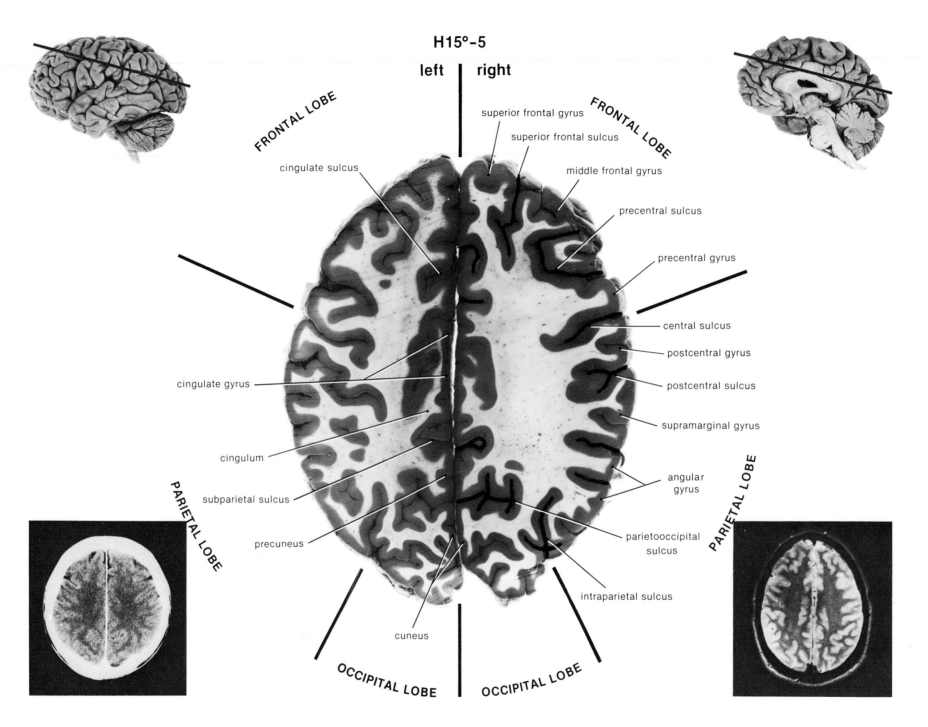

H15°-5

left | right

FRONTAL LOBE

FRONTAL LOBE

superior frontal gyrus

superior frontal sulcus

middle frontal gyrus

precentral sulcus

precentral gyrus

central sulcus

postcentral gyrus

postcentral sulcus

supramarginal gyrus

angular gyrus

parietooccipital sulcus

intraparietal sulcus

cingulate sulcus

cingulate gyrus

cingulum

subparietal sulcus

precuneus

cuneus

PARIETAL LOBE

PARIETAL LOBE

OCCIPITAL LOBE

OCCIPITAL LOBE

150

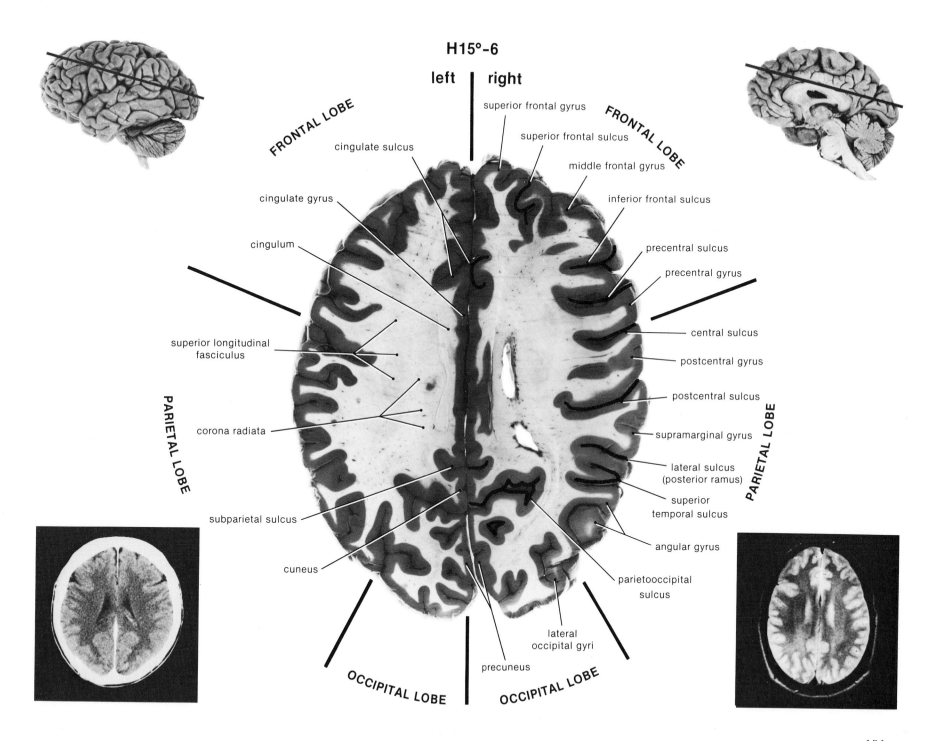

H15°-6

left | right

FRONTAL LOBE

FRONTAL LOBE

superior frontal gyrus

superior frontal sulcus

middle frontal gyrus

inferior frontal sulcus

cingulate sulcus

cingulate gyrus

cingulum

precentral sulcus

precentral gyrus

central sulcus

postcentral gyrus

superior longitudinal fasciculus

postcentral sulcus

supramarginal gyrus

corona radiata

lateral sulcus (posterior ramus)

superior temporal sulcus

PARIETAL LOBE

PARIETAL LOBE

angular gyrus

subparietal sulcus

parietooccipital sulcus

cuneus

lateral occipital gyri

precuneus

OCCIPITAL LOBE

OCCIPITAL LOBE

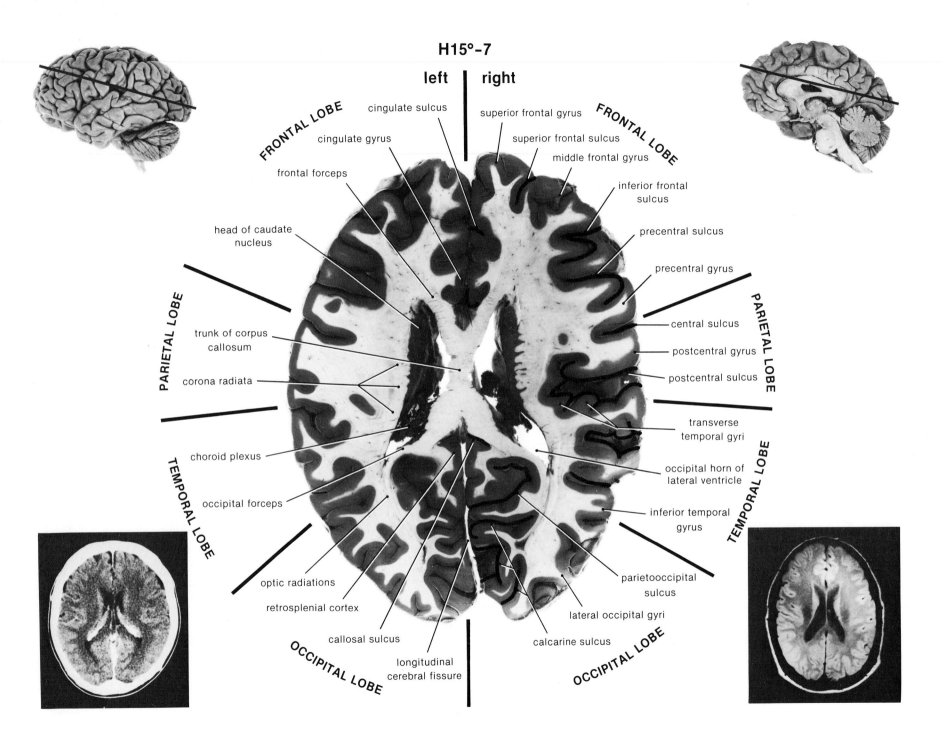

H15°-7

left | right

FRONTAL LOBE

cingulate sulcus
cingulate gyrus
frontal forceps
head of caudate nucleus

superior frontal gyrus
superior frontal sulcus
middle frontal gyrus
inferior frontal sulcus
precentral sulcus
precentral gyrus

FRONTAL LOBE

PARIETAL LOBE

trunk of corpus callosum
corona radiata
choroid plexus
occipital forceps

central sulcus
postcentral gyrus
postcentral sulcus
transverse temporal gyri
occipital horn of lateral ventricle
inferior temporal gyrus

PARIETAL LOBE

TEMPORAL LOBE

optic radiations
retrosplenial cortex
callosal sulcus
longitudinal cerebral fissure

parietooccipital sulcus
lateral occipital gyri
calcarine sulcus

TEMPORAL LOBE

OCCIPITAL LOBE

OCCIPITAL LOBE

152

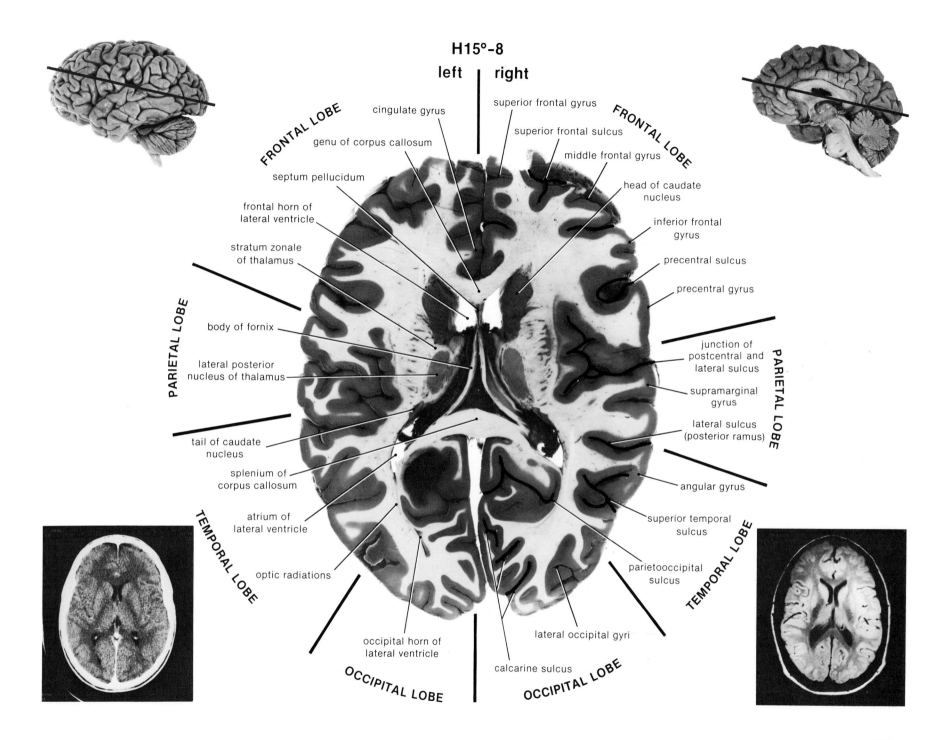

H15°-8

left | right

FRONTAL LOBE

cingulate gyrus

genu of corpus callosum

septum pellucidum

frontal horn of lateral ventricle

stratum zonale of thalamus

PARIETAL LOBE

body of fornix

lateral posterior nucleus of thalamus

tail of caudate nucleus

splenium of corpus callosum

atrium of lateral ventricle

optic radiations

TEMPORAL LOBE

occipital horn of lateral ventricle

OCCIPITAL LOBE

superior frontal gyrus

superior frontal sulcus

middle frontal gyrus

FRONTAL LOBE

head of caudate nucleus

inferior frontal gyrus

precentral sulcus

precentral gyrus

junction of postcentral and lateral sulcus

PARIETAL LOBE

supramarginal gyrus

lateral sulcus (posterior ramus)

angular gyrus

superior temporal sulcus

parietooccipital sulcus

TEMPORAL LOBE

lateral occipital gyri

calcarine sulcus

OCCIPITAL LOBE

153

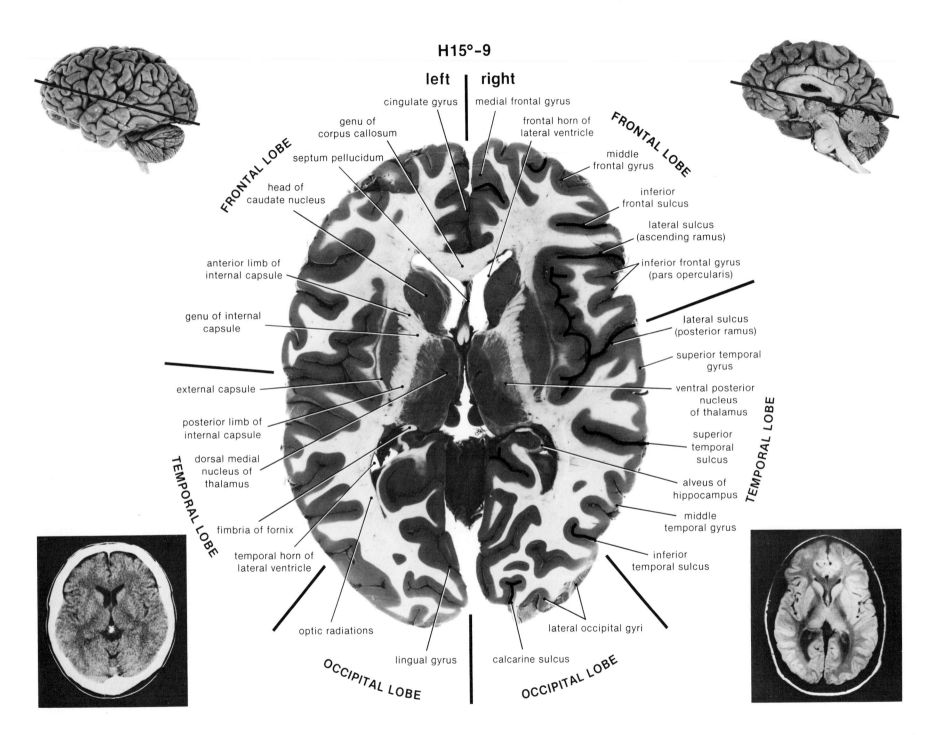

H15°-9

left | right

FRONTAL LOBE

cingulate gyrus
medial frontal gyrus
genu of corpus callosum
frontal horn of lateral ventricle
FRONTAL LOBE
septum pellucidum
middle frontal gyrus
head of caudate nucleus
inferior frontal sulcus
lateral sulcus (ascending ramus)
anterior limb of internal capsule
inferior frontal gyrus (pars opercularis)
genu of internal capsule
lateral sulcus (posterior ramus)
superior temporal gyrus
external capsule
ventral posterior nucleus of thalamus
posterior limb of internal capsule
superior temporal sulcus
dorsal medial nucleus of thalamus
TEMPORAL LOBE
alveus of hippocampus
fimbria of fornix
middle temporal gyrus
temporal horn of lateral ventricle
inferior temporal sulcus
TEMPORAL LOBE
optic radiations
lateral occipital gyri
lingual gyrus
calcarine sulcus
OCCIPITAL LOBE
OCCIPITAL LOBE

154

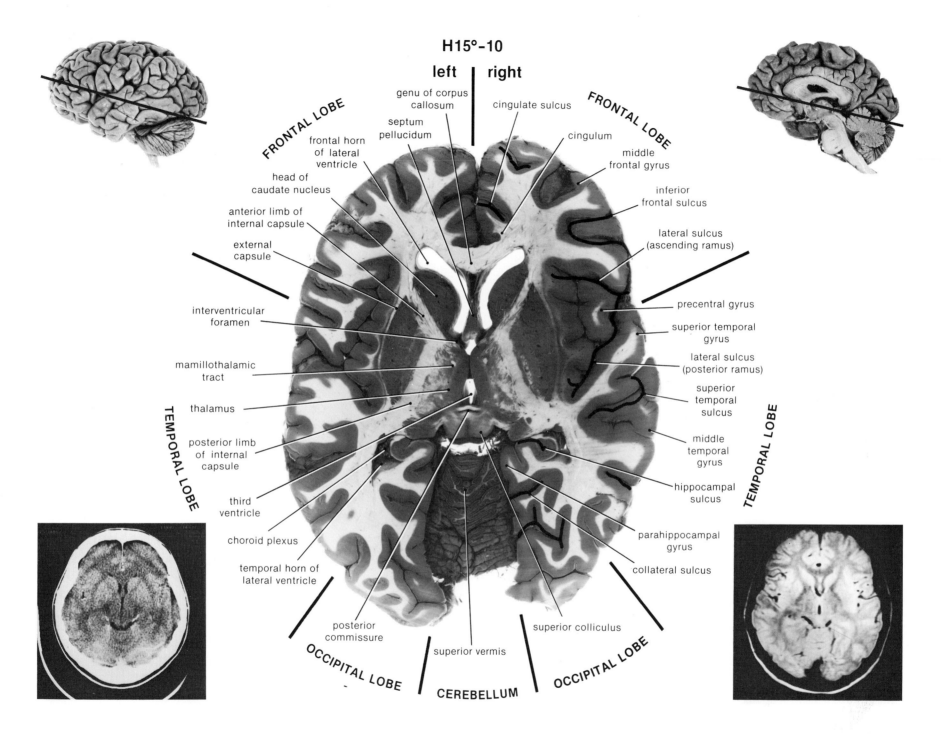

H15°-10

left | right

FRONTAL LOBE

genu of corpus callosum

cingulate sulcus

septum pellucidum

cingulum

frontal horn of lateral ventricle

FRONTAL LOBE

middle frontal gyrus

head of caudate nucleus

inferior frontal sulcus

anterior limb of internal capsule

lateral sulcus (ascending ramus)

external capsule

precentral gyrus

interventricular foramen

superior temporal gyrus

lateral sulcus (posterior ramus)

mamillothalamic tract

superior temporal sulcus

TEMPORAL LOBE

thalamus

middle temporal gyrus

posterior limb of internal capsule

TEMPORAL LOBE

third ventricle

hippocampal sulcus

choroid plexus

parahippocampal gyrus

temporal horn of lateral ventricle

collateral sulcus

posterior commissure

superior colliculus

OCCIPITAL LOBE

superior vermis

OCCIPITAL LOBE

CEREBELLUM

155

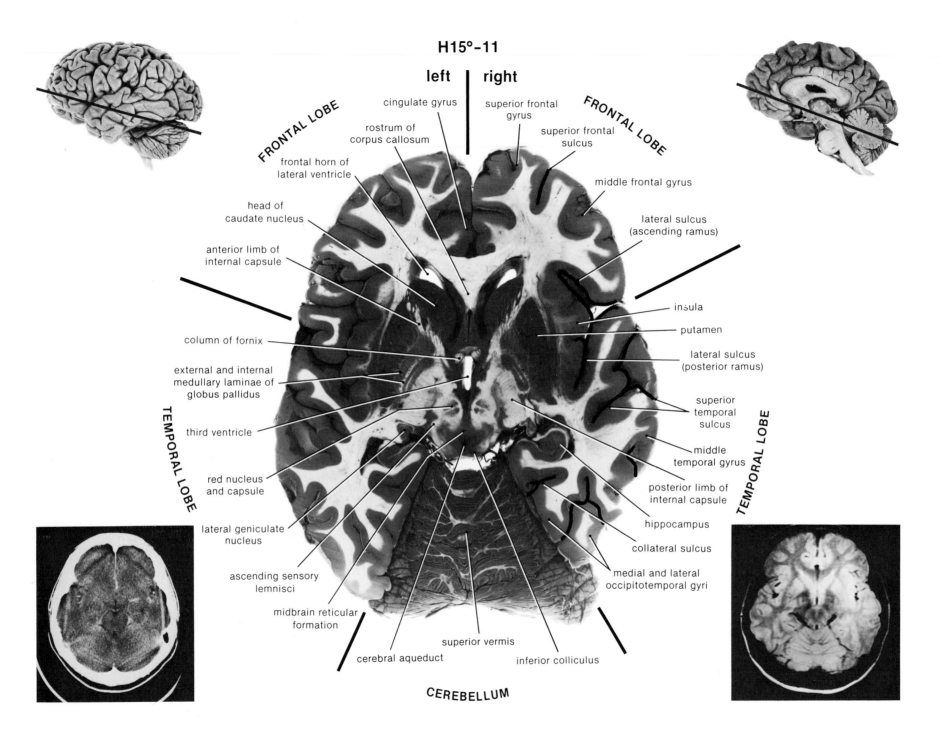

left   right

FRONTAL LOBE   **FRONTAL LOBE**

cingulate gyrus

superior frontal gyrus

rostrum of corpus callosum

superior frontal sulcus

frontal horn of lateral ventricle

middle frontal gyrus

head of caudate nucleus

lateral sulcus (ascending ramus)

anterior limb of internal capsule

insula

putamen

column of fornix

lateral sulcus (posterior ramus)

external and internal medullary laminae of globus pallidus

superior temporal sulcus

third ventricle

middle temporal gyrus

red nucleus and capsule

posterior limb of internal capsule

hippocampus

lateral geniculate nucleus

collateral sulcus

ascending sensory lemnisci

medial and lateral occipitotemporal gyri

midbrain reticular formation

cerebral aqueduct   superior vermis   inferior colliculus

TEMPORAL LOBE   **TEMPORAL LOBE**

CEREBELLUM

156

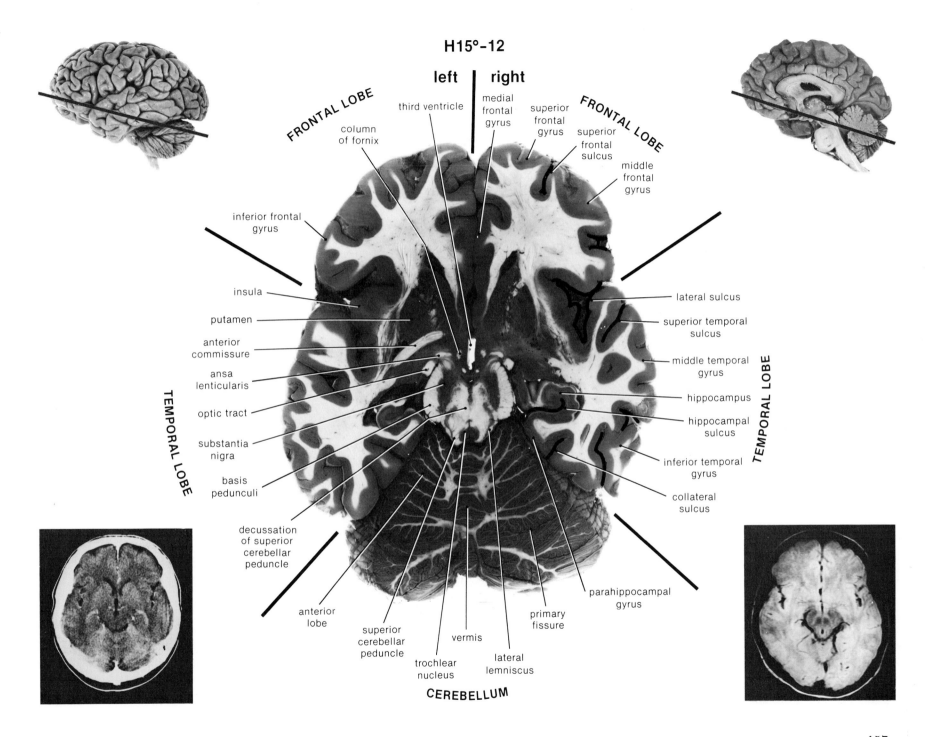

left right

FRONTAL LOBE

third ventricle

medial frontal gyrus

superior frontal gyrus

FRONTAL LOBE

superior frontal sulcus

column of fornix

middle frontal gyrus

inferior frontal gyrus

lateral sulcus

insula

superior temporal sulcus

putamen

middle temporal gyrus

anterior commissure

hippocampus

ansa lenticularis

hippocampal sulcus

optic tract

TEMPORAL LOBE

substantia nigra

inferior temporal gyrus

basis pedunculi

collateral sulcus

TEMPORAL LOBE

decussation of superior cerebellar peduncle

parahippocampal gyrus

anterior lobe

superior cerebellar peduncle

vermis

primary fissure

trochlear nucleus

lateral lemniscus

CEREBELLUM

157

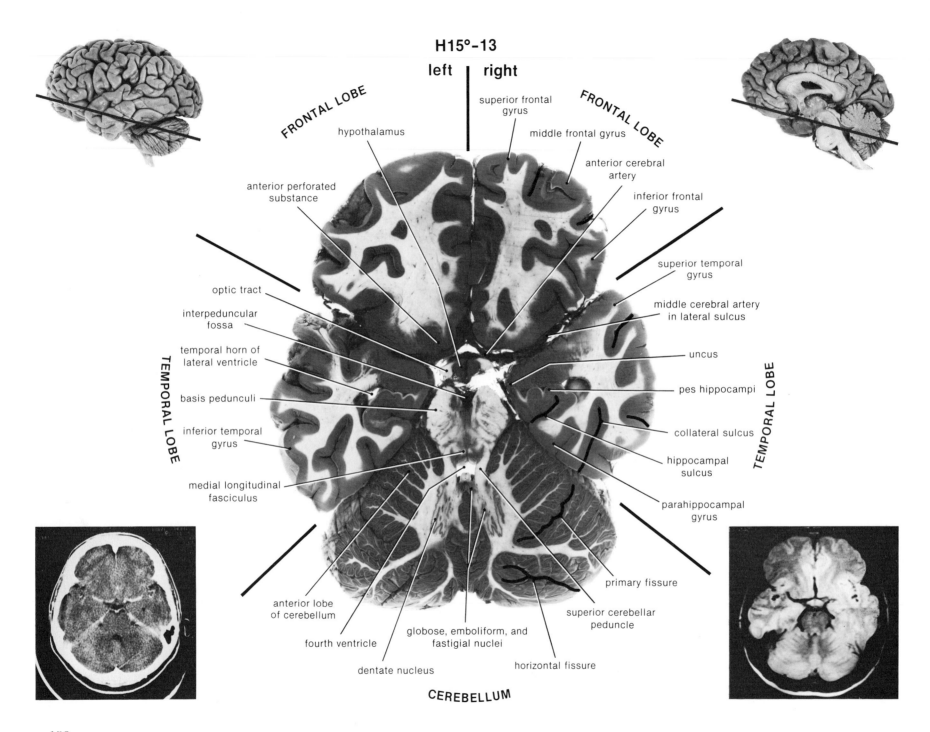

H15°-13

left | right

FRONTAL LOBE

FRONTAL LOBE

TEMPORAL LOBE

TEMPORAL LOBE

CEREBELLUM

- superior frontal gyrus
- middle frontal gyrus
- anterior cerebral artery
- inferior frontal gyrus
- superior temporal gyrus
- middle cerebral artery in lateral sulcus
- uncus
- pes hippocampi
- collateral sulcus
- hippocampal sulcus
- parahippocampal gyrus
- primary fissure
- superior cerebellar peduncle
- horizontal fissure
- dentate nucleus
- globose, emboliform, and fastigial nuclei
- fourth ventricle
- anterior lobe of cerebellum
- medial longitudinal fasciculus
- inferior temporal gyrus
- basis pedunculi
- temporal horn of lateral ventricle
- interpeduncular fossa
- optic tract
- anterior perforated substance
- hypothalamus

158

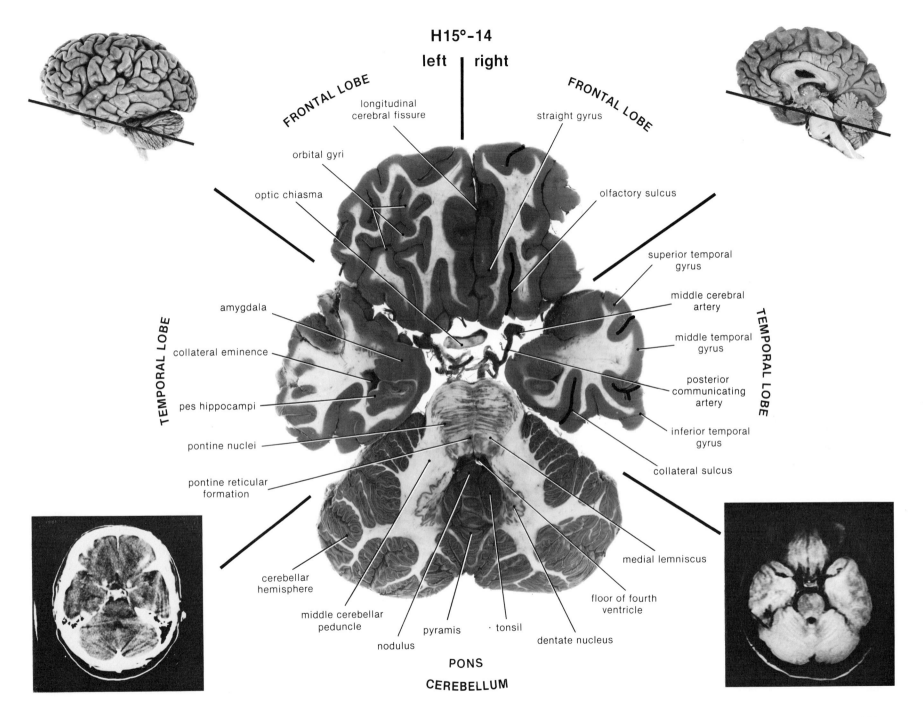

FRONTAL LOBE

longitudinal cerebral fissure

straight gyrus

orbital gyri

olfactory sulcus

optic chiasma

FRONTAL LOBE

superior temporal gyrus

middle cerebral artery

amygdala

middle temporal gyrus

collateral eminence

posterior communicating artery

TEMPORAL LOBE

pes hippocampi

inferior temporal gyrus

pontine nuclei

TEMPORAL LOBE

pontine reticular formation

collateral sulcus

medial lemniscus

cerebellar hemisphere

middle cerebellar peduncle

floor of fourth ventricle

nodulus

pyramis

tonsil

dentate nucleus

PONS

CEREBELLUM

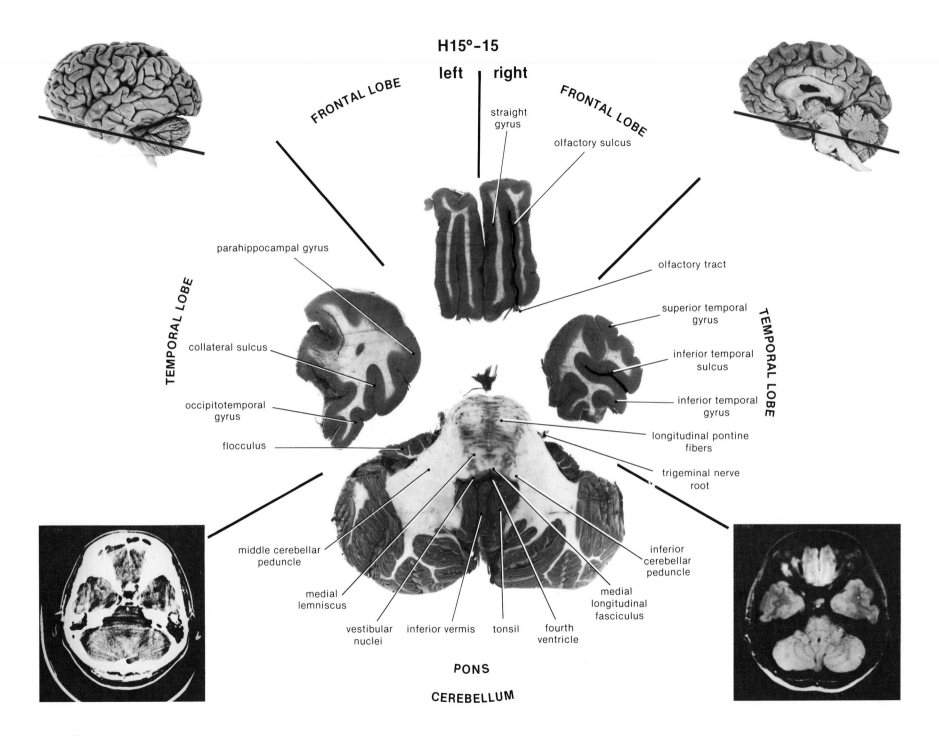

H15°-15

left | right

FRONTAL LOBE

FRONTAL LOBE

straight gyrus

olfactory sulcus

parahippocampal gyrus

olfactory tract

TEMPORAL LOBE

TEMPORAL LOBE

superior temporal gyrus

collateral sulcus

inferior temporal sulcus

occipitotemporal gyrus

inferior temporal gyrus

flocculus

longitudinal pontine fibers

trigeminal nerve root

middle cerebellar peduncle

inferior cerebellar peduncle

medial lemniscus

medial longitudinal fasciculus

vestibular nuclei

inferior vermis

tonsil

fourth ventricle

PONS

CEREBELLUM

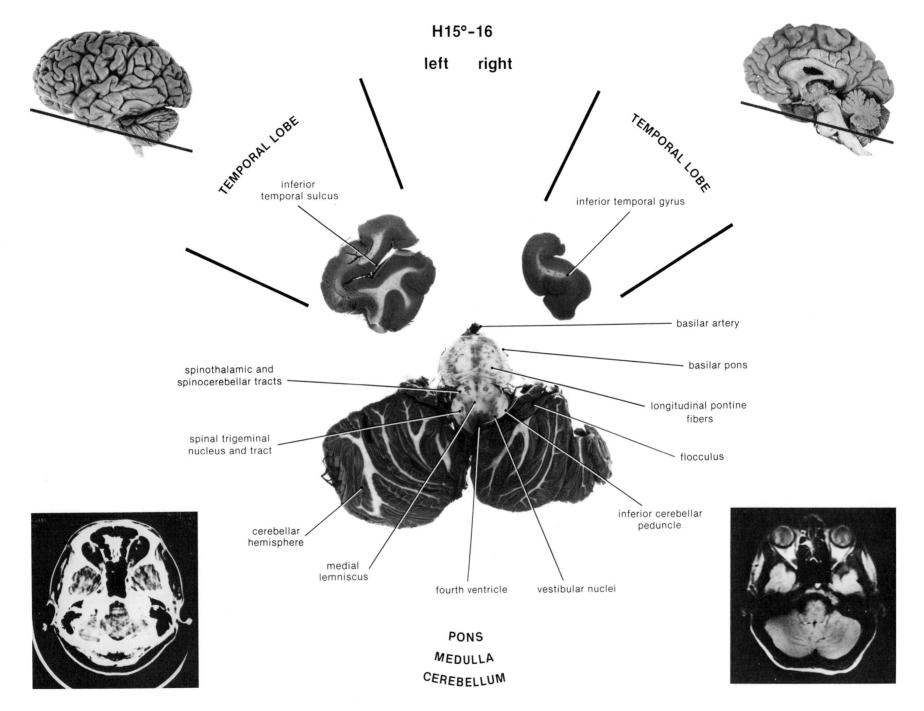

left   right

TEMPORAL LOBE

inferior
temporal sulcus

TEMPORAL LOBE

inferior temporal gyrus

basilar artery

basilar pons

spinothalamic and
spinocerebellar tracts

longitudinal pontine
fibers

spinal trigeminal
nucleus and tract

flocculus

inferior cerebellar
peduncle

cerebellar
hemisphere

medial
lemniscus

fourth ventricle

vestibular nuclei

PONS

MEDULLA

CEREBELLUM

161

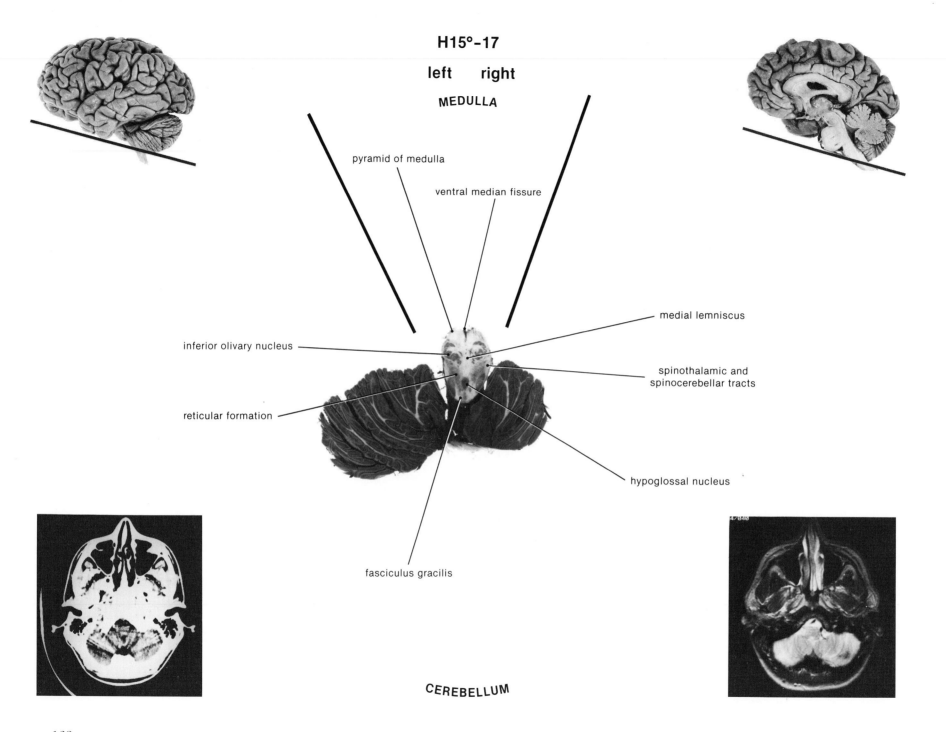

H15°–17

left   right

MEDULLA

pyramid of medulla

ventral median fissure

medial lemniscus

inferior olivary nucleus

spinothalamic and
spinocerebellar tracts

reticular formation

hypoglossal nucleus

fasciculus gracilis

CEREBELLUM

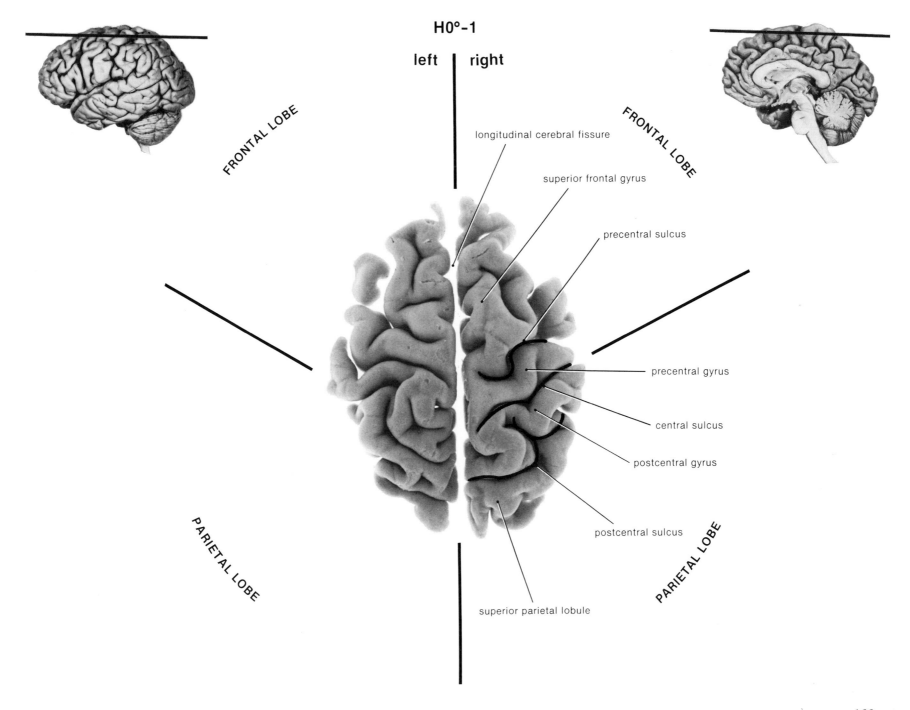

left | right

FRONTAL LOBE

FRONTAL LOBE

longitudinal cerebral fissure

superior frontal gyrus

precentral sulcus

precentral gyrus

central sulcus

postcentral gyrus

postcentral sulcus

PARIETAL LOBE

PARIETAL LOBE

superior parietal lobule

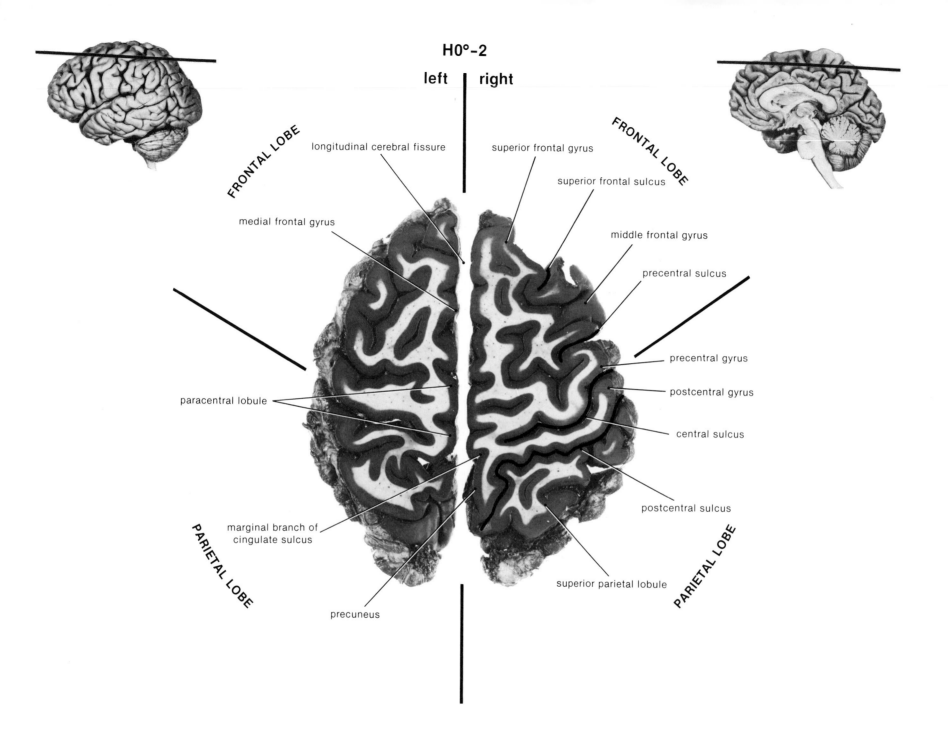

left | right

FRONTAL LOBE

FRONTAL LOBE

longitudinal cerebral fissure

superior frontal gyrus

superior frontal sulcus

medial frontal gyrus

middle frontal gyrus

precentral sulcus

precentral gyrus

postcentral gyrus

paracentral lobule

central sulcus

postcentral sulcus

marginal branch of cingulate sulcus

PARIETAL LOBE

PARIETAL LOBE

superior parietal lobule

precuneus

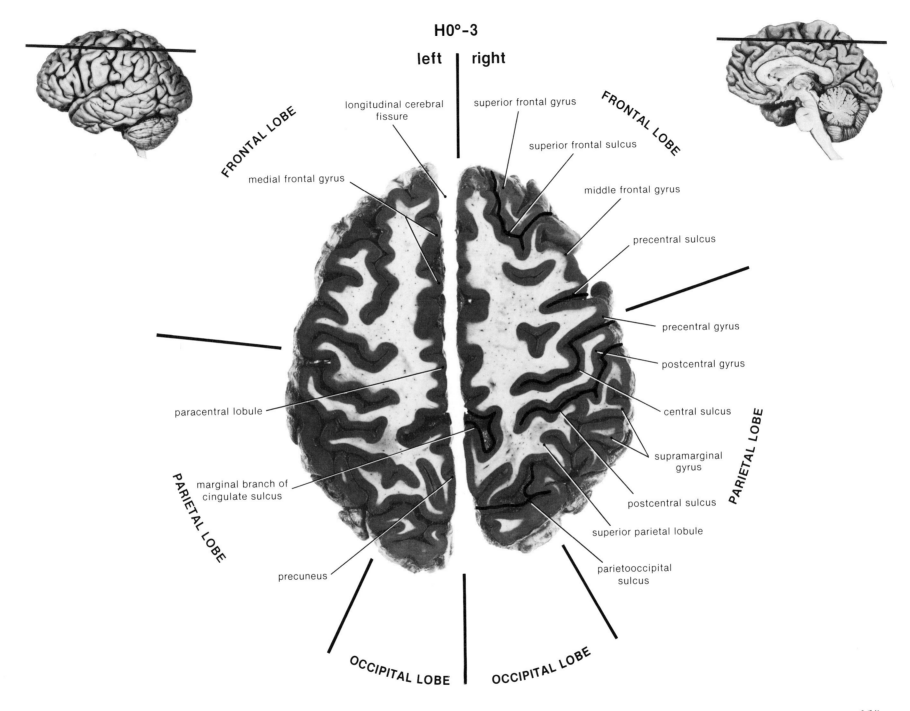

H0°-3

left | right

FRONTAL LOBE

FRONTAL LOBE

FRONTAL LOBE

longitudinal cerebral fissure

superior frontal gyrus

superior frontal sulcus

medial frontal gyrus

middle frontal gyrus

precentral sulcus

precentral gyrus

postcentral gyrus

paracentral lobule

central sulcus

supramarginal gyrus

PARIETAL LOBE

postcentral sulcus

marginal branch of cingulate sulcus

superior parietal lobule

PARIETAL LOBE

parietooccipital sulcus

precuneus

OCCIPITAL LOBE

OCCIPITAL LOBE

165

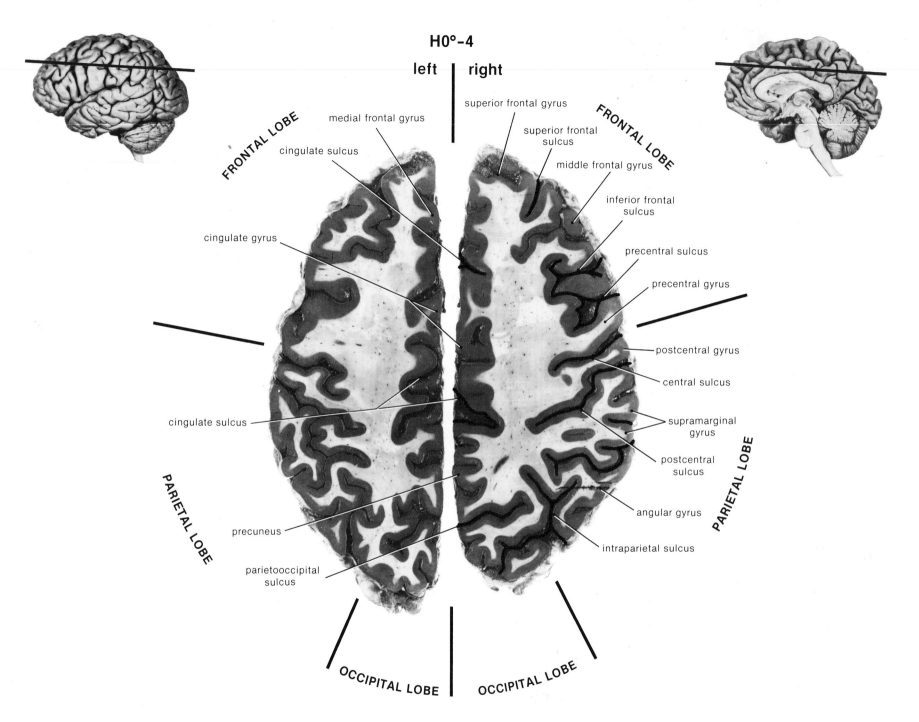

H0°-4

left | right

FRONTAL LOBE

superior frontal gyrus

medial frontal gyrus

superior frontal sulcus

cingulate sulcus

FRONTAL LOBE

middle frontal gyrus

inferior frontal sulcus

cingulate gyrus

precentral sulcus

precentral gyrus

postcentral gyrus

central sulcus

cingulate sulcus

supramarginal gyrus

PARIETAL LOBE

postcentral sulcus

precuneus

angular gyrus

PARIETAL LOBE

parietooccipital sulcus

intraparietal sulcus

OCCIPITAL LOBE | OCCIPITAL LOBE

166

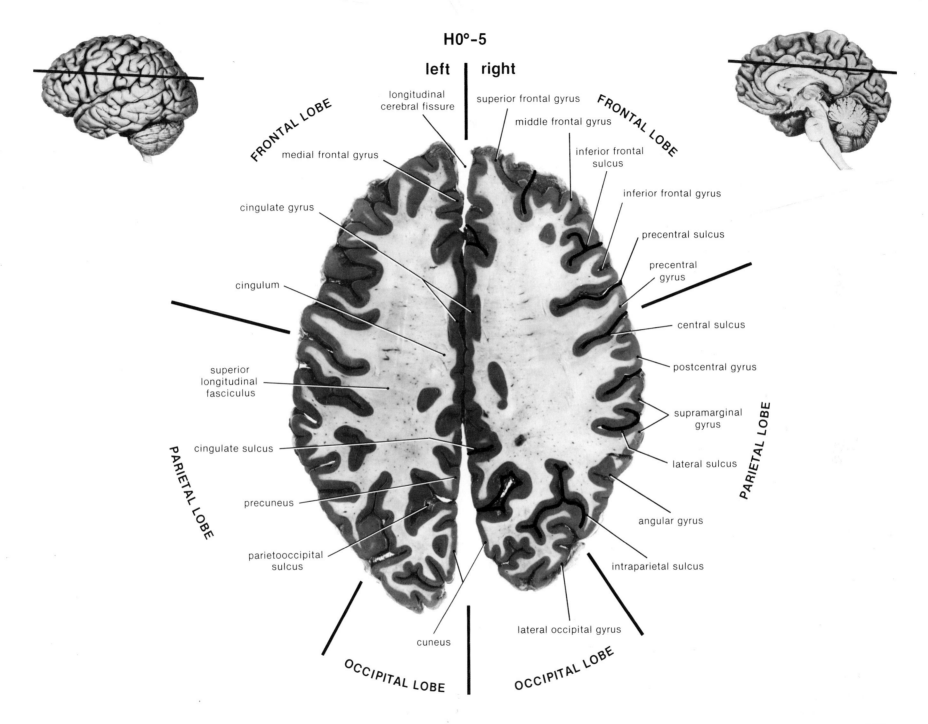

H0°-5

left | **right**

FRONTAL LOBE

longitudinal cerebral fissure

superior frontal gyrus

FRONTAL LOBE

middle frontal gyrus

medial frontal gyrus

inferior frontal sulcus

cingulate gyrus

inferior frontal gyrus

precentral sulcus

cingulum

precentral gyrus

central sulcus

superior longitudinal fasciculus

postcentral gyrus

supramarginal gyrus

PARIETAL LOBE

PARIETAL LOBE

cingulate sulcus

lateral sulcus

precuneus

angular gyrus

parietooccipital sulcus

intraparietal sulcus

cuneus

lateral occipital gyrus

OCCIPITAL LOBE

OCCIPITAL LOBE

167

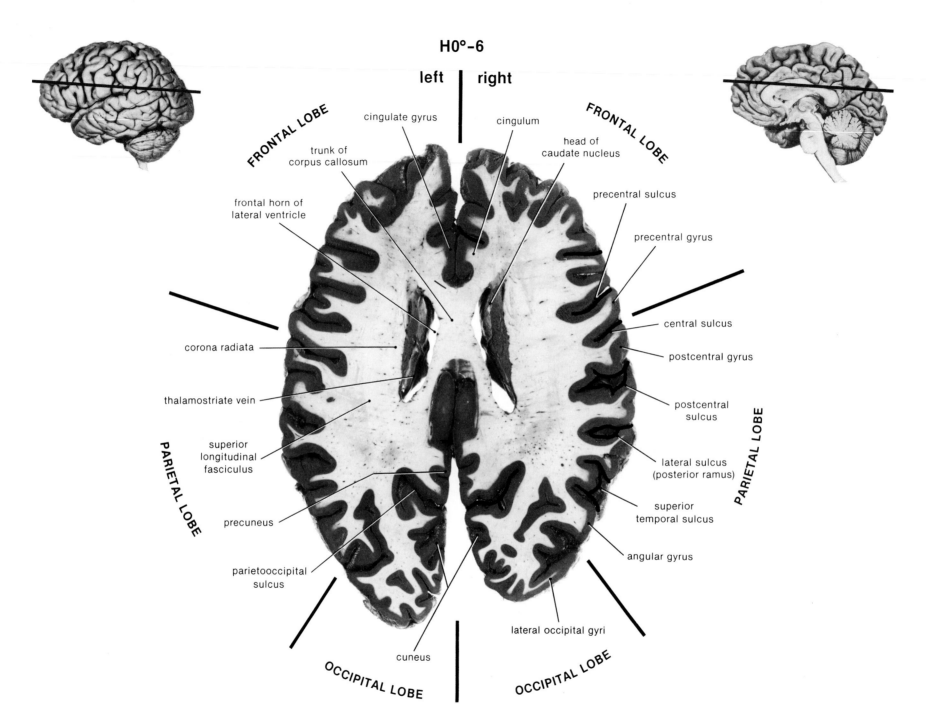

H0°-6

left | right

FRONTAL LOBE

FRONTAL LOBE

cingulate gyrus

cingulum

head of caudate nucleus

trunk of corpus callosum

precentral sulcus

precentral gyrus

frontal horn of lateral ventricle

central sulcus

postcentral gyrus

corona radiata

thalamostriate vein

postcentral sulcus

superior longitudinal fasciculus

PARIETAL LOBE

lateral sulcus (posterior ramus)

PARIETAL LOBE

precuneus

superior temporal sulcus

angular gyrus

parietooccipital sulcus

lateral occipital gyri

cuneus

OCCIPITAL LOBE

OCCIPITAL LOBE

168

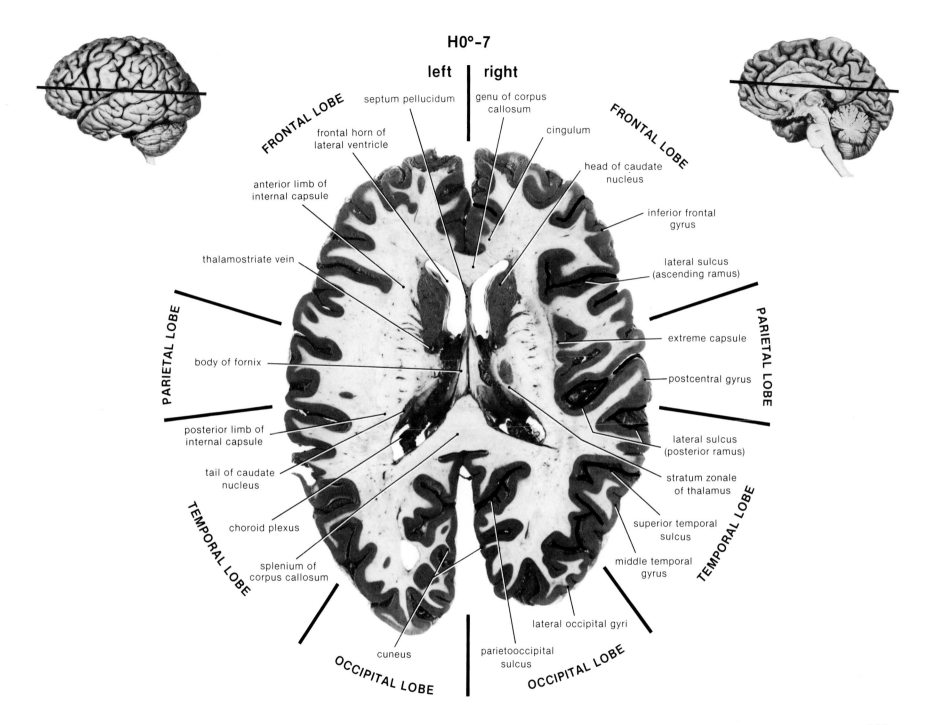

H0°-7

left | right

FRONTAL LOBE

septum pellucidum

genu of corpus callosum

FRONTAL LOBE

frontal horn of lateral ventricle

cingulum

head of caudate nucleus

anterior limb of internal capsule

inferior frontal gyrus

thalamostriate vein

lateral sulcus (ascending ramus)

PARIETAL LOBE

PARIETAL LOBE

extreme capsule

body of fornix

postcentral gyrus

posterior limb of internal capsule

lateral sulcus (posterior ramus)

tail of caudate nucleus

stratum zonale of thalamus

choroid plexus

superior temporal sulcus

TEMPORAL LOBE

middle temporal gyrus

TEMPORAL LOBE

splenium of corpus callosum

lateral occipital gyri

cuneus

parietooccipital sulcus

OCCIPITAL LOBE

OCCIPITAL LOBE

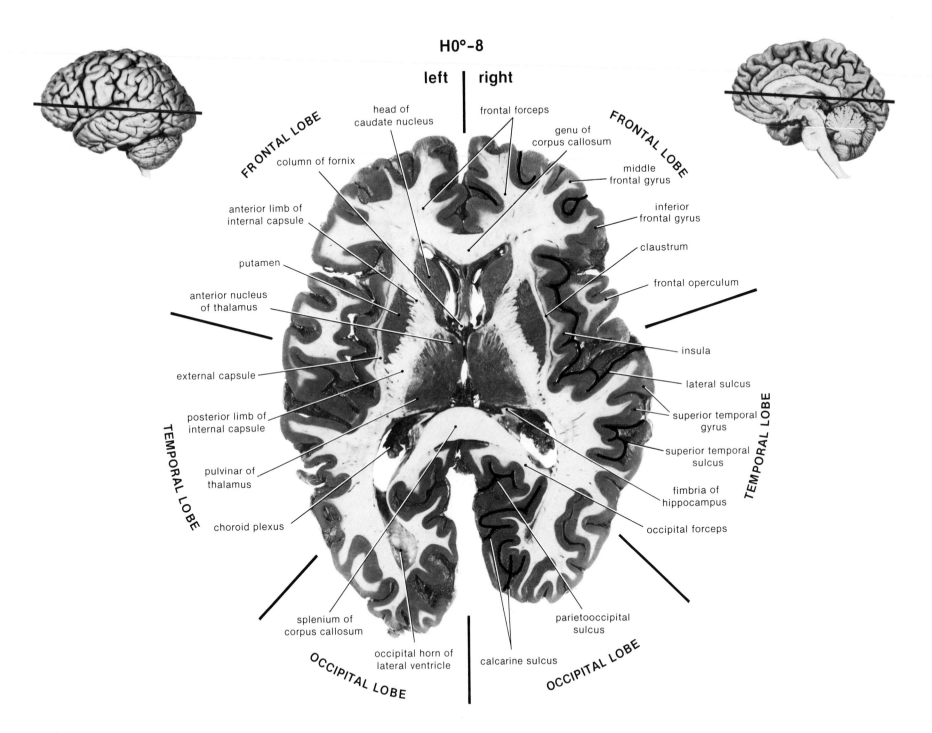

left | right

FRONTAL LOBE

head of
caudate nucleus

frontal forceps

genu of
corpus callosum

FRONTAL LOBE

column of fornix

middle
frontal gyrus

anterior limb of
internal capsule

inferior
frontal gyrus

claustrum

putamen

frontal operculum

anterior nucleus
of thalamus

insula

external capsule

lateral sulcus

superior temporal
gyrus

posterior limb of
internal capsule

superior temporal
sulcus

TEMPORAL LOBE

pulvinar of
thalamus

fimbria of
hippocampus

TEMPORAL LOBE

choroid plexus

occipital forceps

splenium of
corpus callosum

parietooccipital
sulcus

occipital horn of
lateral ventricle

calcarine sulcus

OCCIPITAL LOBE

OCCIPITAL LOBE

170

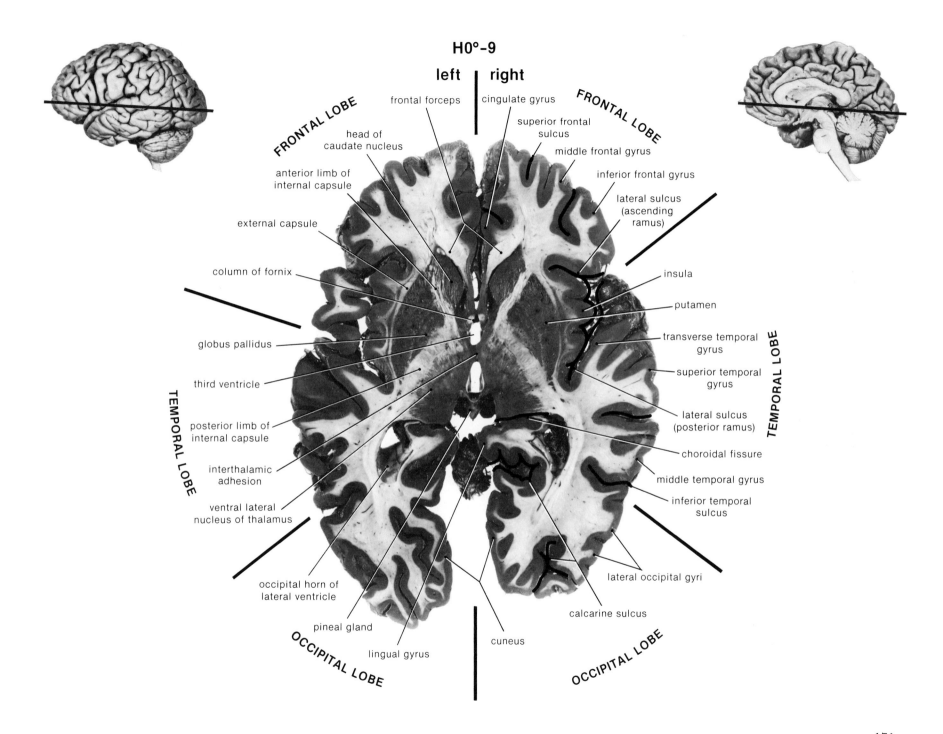

left | **right**

FRONTAL LOBE

frontal forceps

cingulate gyrus

FRONTAL LOBE

head of caudate nucleus

superior frontal sulcus

anterior limb of internal capsule

middle frontal gyrus

inferior frontal gyrus

external capsule

lateral sulcus (ascending ramus)

column of fornix

insula

putamen

globus pallidus

transverse temporal gyrus

third ventricle

superior temporal gyrus

TEMPORAL LOBE

posterior limb of internal capsule

lateral sulcus (posterior ramus)

interthalamic adhesion

choroidal fissure

TEMPORAL LOBE

ventral lateral nucleus of thalamus

middle temporal gyrus

inferior temporal sulcus

occipital horn of lateral ventricle

lateral occipital gyri

pineal gland

calcarine sulcus

lingual gyrus

cuneus

OCCIPITAL LOBE

OCCIPITAL LOBE

171

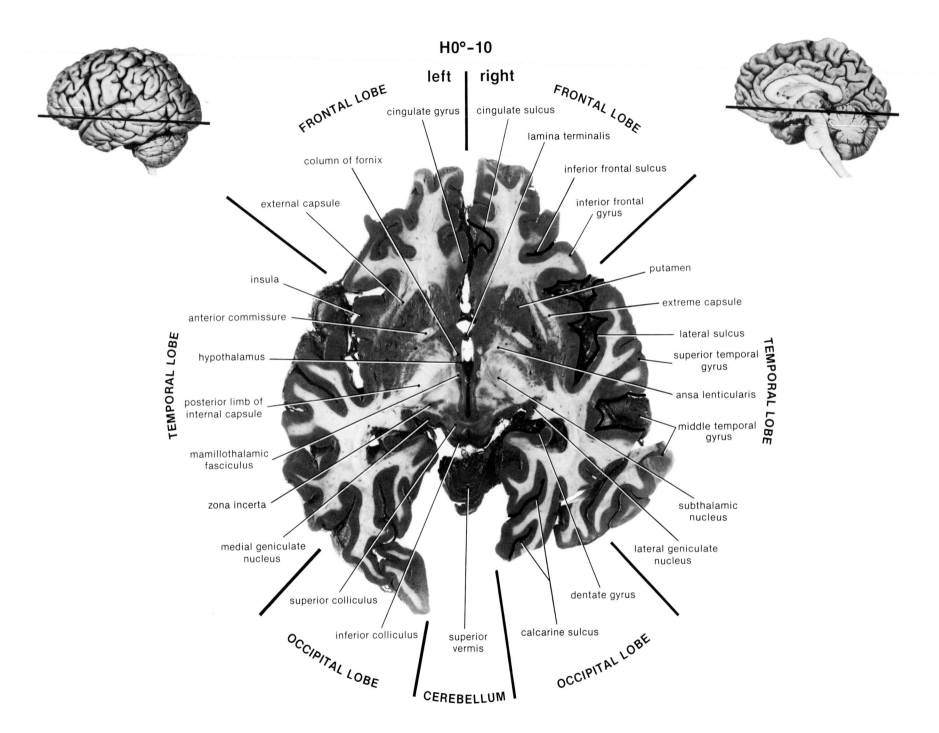

H0°-10

left | right

FRONTAL LOBE

FRONTAL LOBE

cingulate gyrus
cingulate sulcus
lamina terminalis
column of fornix
inferior frontal sulcus
inferior frontal gyrus
external capsule
putamen
insula
extreme capsule
anterior commissure
lateral sulcus
superior temporal gyrus
hypothalamus
ansa lenticularis
posterior limb of internal capsule
mamillothalamic fasciculus
middle temporal gyrus
zona incerta
subthalamic nucleus
medial geniculate nucleus
lateral geniculate nucleus
superior colliculus
dentate gyrus
inferior colliculus
superior vermis
calcarine sulcus

TEMPORAL LOBE

TEMPORAL LOBE

OCCIPITAL LOBE

OCCIPITAL LOBE

CEREBELLUM

172

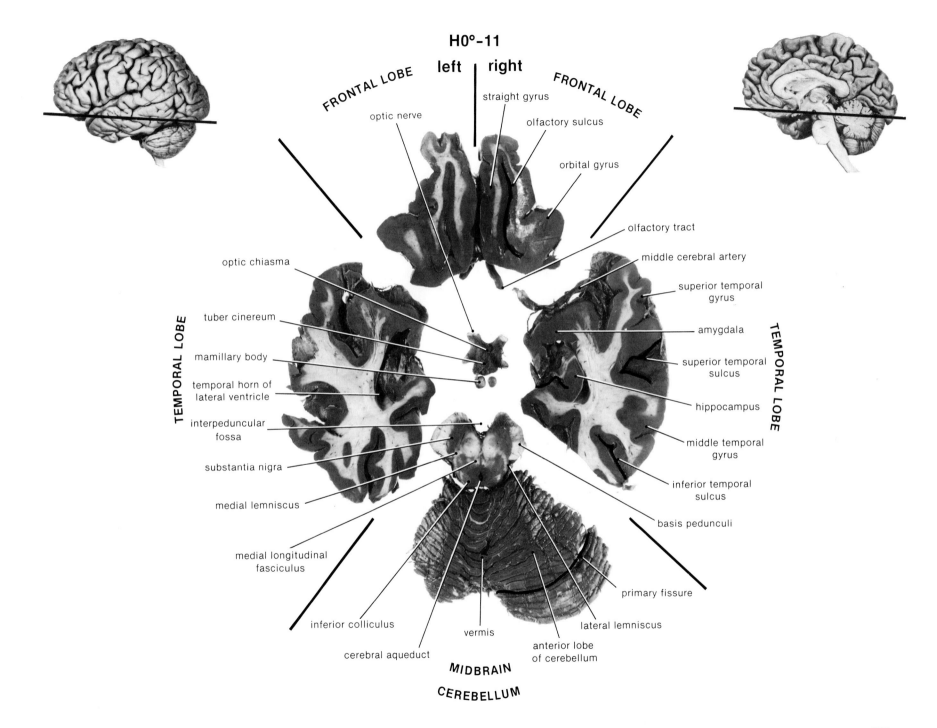

H0°-11

left | right

FRONTAL LOBE

FRONTAL LOBE

straight gyrus

optic nerve

olfactory sulcus

orbital gyrus

olfactory tract

middle cerebral artery

optic chiasma

superior temporal gyrus

tuber cinereum

amygdala

mamillary body

superior temporal sulcus

TEMPORAL LOBE

temporal horn of lateral ventricle

hippocampus

TEMPORAL LOBE

interpeduncular fossa

middle temporal gyrus

substantia nigra

inferior temporal sulcus

medial lemniscus

basis pedunculi

medial longitudinal fasciculus

primary fissure

inferior colliculus

lateral lemniscus

vermis

cerebral aqueduct

anterior lobe of cerebellum

MIDBRAIN

CEREBELLUM

173

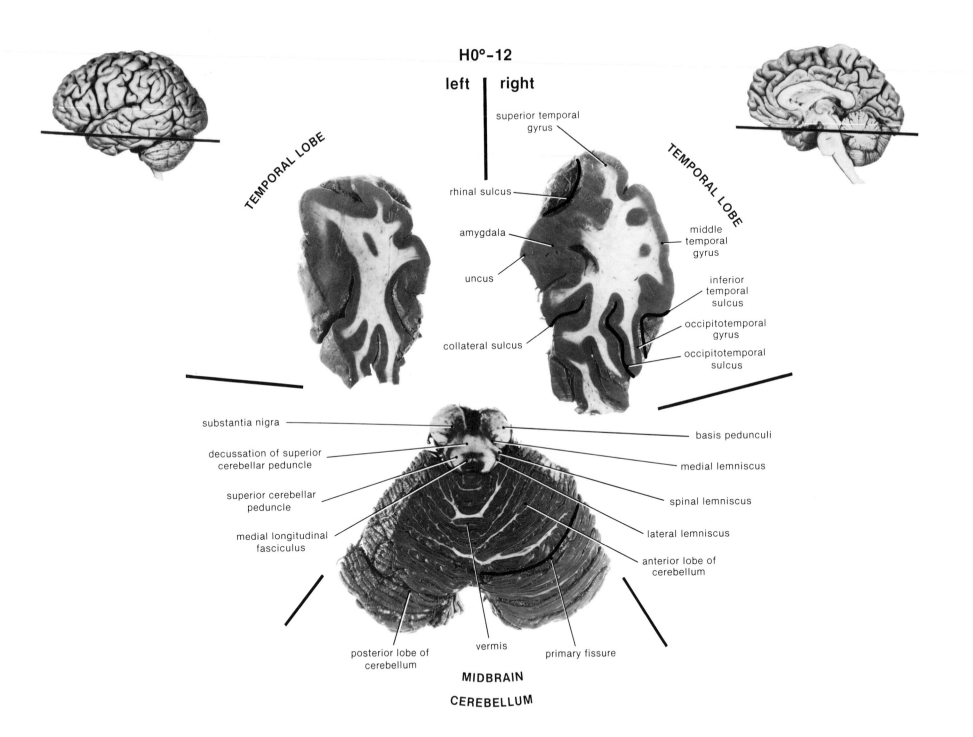

H0°-12

left | right

TEMPORAL LOBE

TEMPORAL LOBE

superior temporal gyrus

rhinal sulcus

amygdala

uncus

collateral sulcus

middle temporal gyrus

inferior temporal sulcus

occipitotemporal gyrus

occipitotemporal sulcus

substantia nigra

decussation of superior cerebellar peduncle

superior cerebellar peduncle

medial longitudinal fasciculus

basis pedunculi

medial lemniscus

spinal lemniscus

lateral lemniscus

anterior lobe of cerebellum

posterior lobe of cerebellum

vermis

primary fissure

MIDBRAIN

CEREBELLUM

174

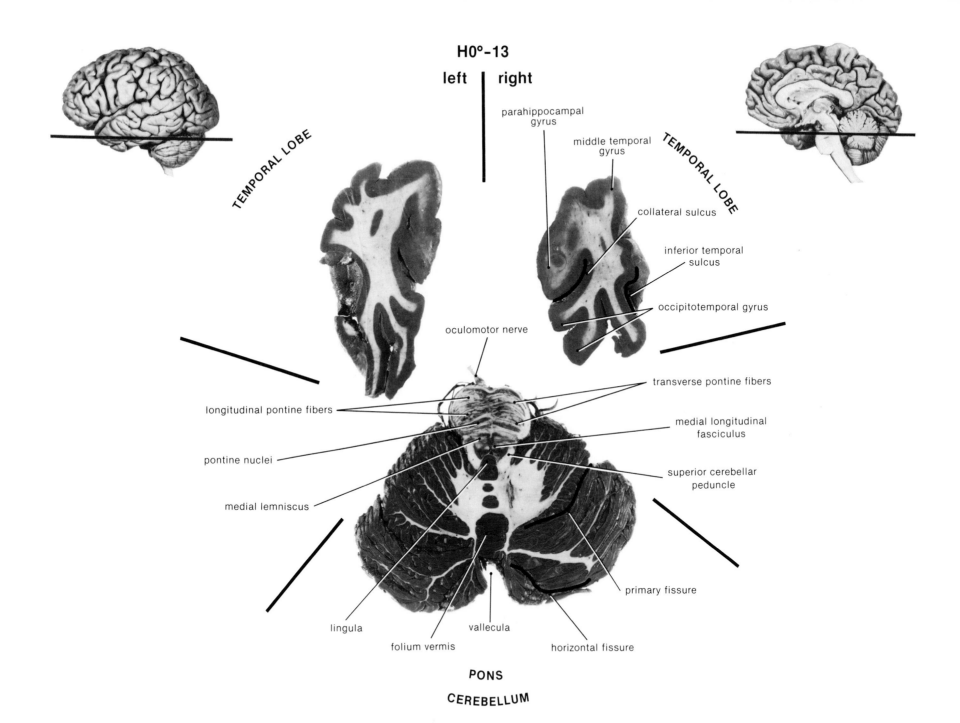

H0°-13

left | right

TEMPORAL LOBE

TEMPORAL LOBE

parahippocampal gyrus

middle temporal gyrus

collateral sulcus

inferior temporal sulcus

occipitotemporal gyrus

oculomotor nerve

transverse pontine fibers

longitudinal pontine fibers

medial longitudinal fasciculus

pontine nuclei

superior cerebellar peduncle

medial lemniscus

primary fissure

lingula

vallecula

folium vermis

horizontal fissure

PONS

CEREBELLUM

175

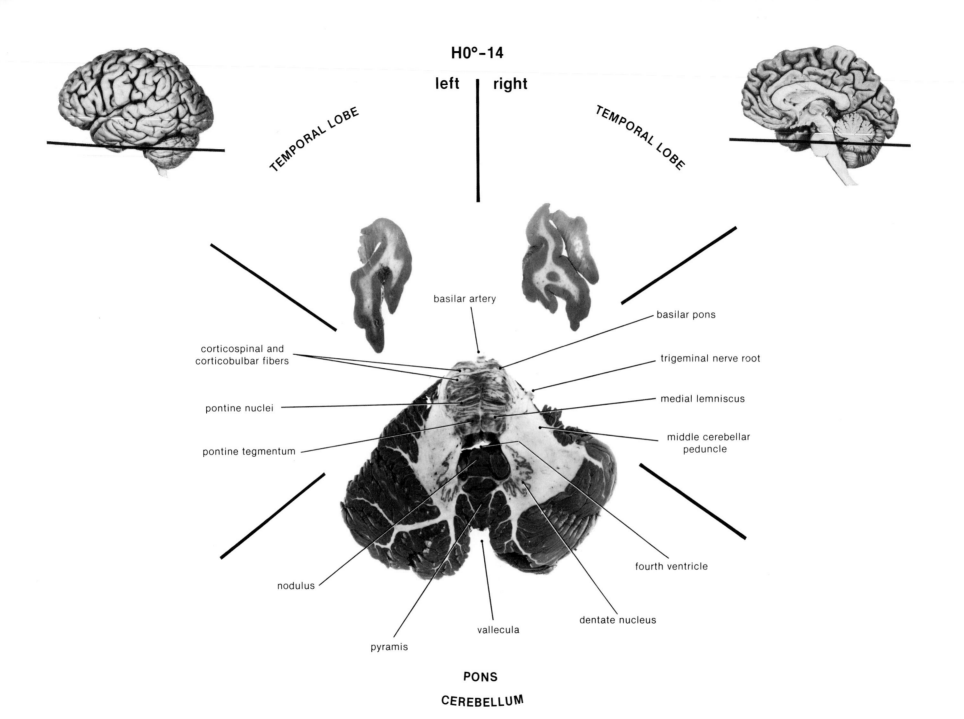

left | right

TEMPORAL LOBE

TEMPORAL LOBE

basilar artery

basilar pons

corticospinal and
corticobulbar fibers

trigeminal nerve root

medial lemniscus

pontine nuclei

middle cerebellar
peduncle

pontine tegmentum

fourth ventricle

nodulus

dentate nucleus

pyramis

vallecula

PONS

CEREBELLUM

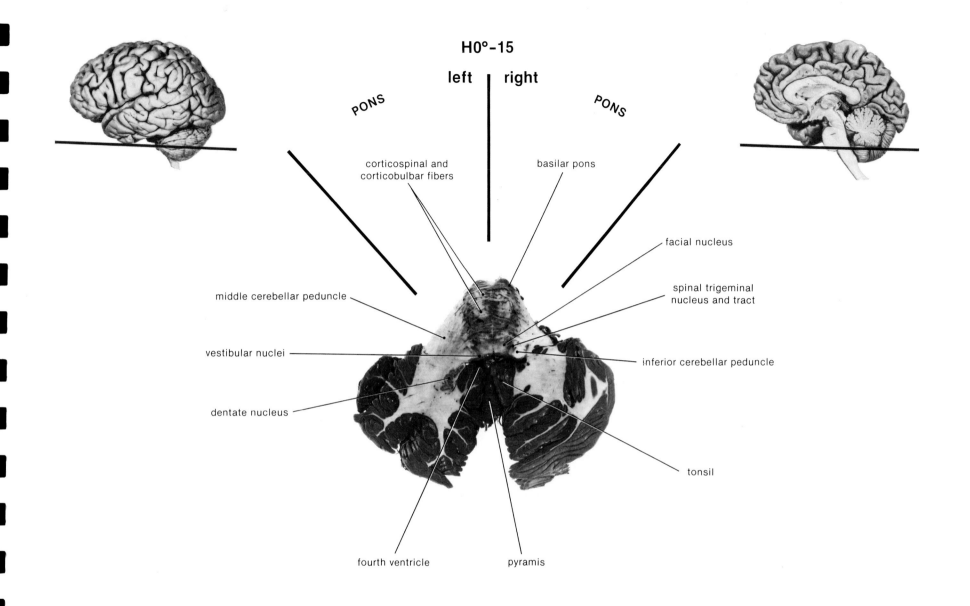

H0°-15

left | right

PONS   PONS

corticospinal and
corticobulbar fibers   basilar pons

facial nucleus

middle cerebellar peduncle   spinal trigeminal
nucleus and tract

vestibular nuclei   inferior cerebellar peduncle

dentate nucleus

tonsil

fourth ventricle   pyramis

CEREBELLUM

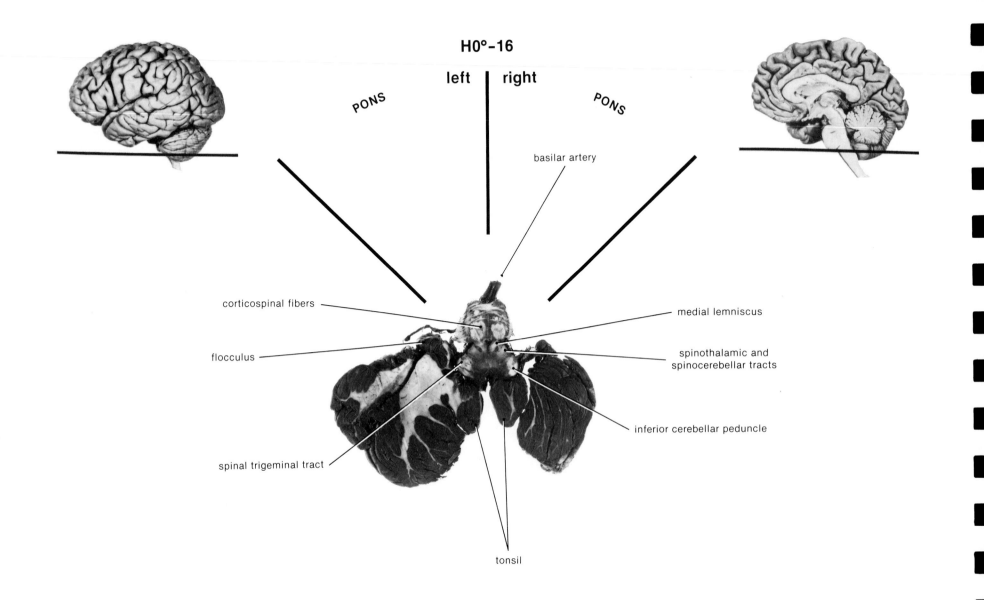

H0°-16

left | right

PONS

PONS

basilar artery

corticospinal fibers

medial lemniscus

flocculus

spinothalamic and spinocerebellar tracts

inferior cerebellar peduncle

spinal trigeminal tract

tonsil

MEDULLA

CEREBELLUM

left | right

MEDULLA

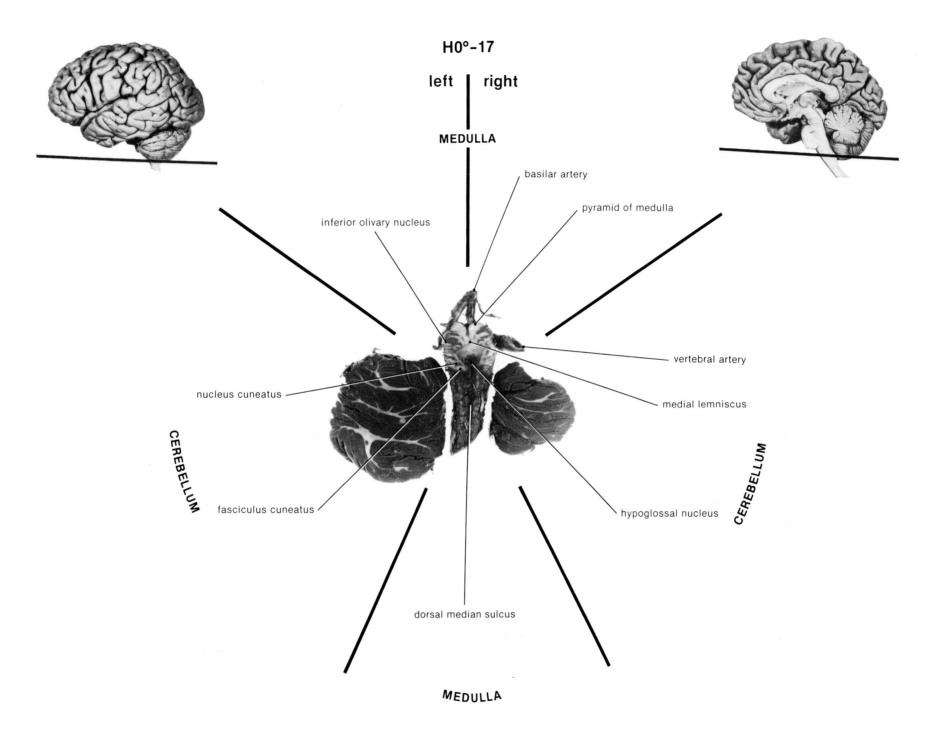

basilar artery

pyramid of medulla

inferior olivary nucleus

vertebral artery

nucleus cuneatus

medial lemniscus

CEREBELLUM

CEREBELLUM

fasciculus cuneatus

hypoglossal nucleus

dorsal median sulcus

MEDULLA

Bibliography

The following are available for purchase through medical bookstores or for reference in libraries:

Barr ML, Kiernan JA: The Human Nervous System: An Anatomical Viewpoint, 4th ed. New York, Harper & Row, 1983.
This is an excellent textbook of neuroanatomy, which is written primarily for medical students and which is used widely in English-speaking medical schools.

Bossy J: Atlas of Neuroanatomy and Special Sense Organs. Philadelphia, WB Saunders Company, 1970.
As the authors state, this is neither a textbook nor a formal manual; it is a teaching and learning aid. It contains innumerable black and white drawings of the structures found in both the central and the peripheral nervous systems.

Brodal A: The Cranial Nerves: Anatomy and Anatomico-Clinical Correlations. Oxford, Blackwell Scientific Publications, 1965.
A classic little book that describes the anatomy, physiology, and clinical correlates of each of the cranial nerves.

Brodal A: Neurological Anatomy in Relation to Clinical Medicine, 3rd ed. New York, Oxford University Press, 1981.
This is a definitive reference textbook of neuroanatomy.

Carpenter MB, Sutin J: Human Neuroananatomy, 8th ed. Baltimore, Williams & Wilkins, 1983.
This long established textbook of neuroanatomy contains many illustrations in color, especially those figures dealing with functional aspects of neuroanatomy.

DeArmond SJ, Fusco MM, Dewey MM: Structure of the Human Brain: A Photographic Atlas, 2nd ed. New York, Oxford University Press, 1976.
This widely used book contains no text. Rather, it is composed of a series of photographs of sections of the brain taken at different planes. The sections are stained for either nuclear material or fiber tracts, and each is accompanied by a well-labeled drawing of the section on the facing page.

FitzGerald MJT: Neuroanatomy Basic and Applied. London, Baillière Tindall, 1985.
This is an excellent new textbook that deals less with the gross morphology of the central nervous system, and more with the functional aspects of neuroananatomy and the clinical sequelae of neurologic disease.

Ford DH, Schadé JP: Atlas of the Human Brain, 2nd ed. New York, Elsevier, 1970.
In addition to a text, this book contains labeled photographs of gross dissections and microscopic sections of the brain.

Frontera JG: Neuroanatomy Laboratory Guide. San Piedras, University of Puerto Rico Press, 1970.
This book contains detailed instructions for dissection of the brain, but the illustrations are black and white line drawings that are heavily labeled. The important structures in the diagrams are indicated, but many of the labels have been purposefully omitted in an attempt to encourage students to label them themselves.

Gluhbegovic N, Williams TH: The Human Brain: A Photographic Guide. New York, Harper & Row, 1980.
This book is neither a text nor a dissection manual. It is a compilation of beautiful photographs (some of which are in monochrome color) of skillfully prepared dissections of the human brain and spinal cord. Each photograph has an accompanying labeled drawing and short descriptive

text on the facing page. No student, and few instructors, would have the skill to prepare the dissections demonstrated in these photographs.

Haines DE: Neuroanatomy: An Atlas of Structures, Sections and Systems. Baltimore, Urban and Schwarzenberg, 1983.
As the title implies, this book contains labeled dissections and sections of the central nervous system as well as line diagrams illustrating functional pathways.

Hall JL, Humberston AO: A Correlative Study Guide for Neuroanatomy, 2nd ed. New York, Harper & Row, 1970.
As the authors state, this book is an adjunct to textbook reading and laboratory sessions in neuroanatomy. It contains a short atlas of the brain and a section of neurological case reports.

Heimer L: The Human Brain and Spinal Cord. New York, Springer-Verlag, 1983.
This book contains a dissection guide to the central nervous system composed of artist's drawings and stained sections in the three basic neuroanatomic planes.

Kiernan JA: Introduction to Human Neurosciences. Philadelphia, J.B. Lippincott, 1987.
This is a scholarly and current book on the structure of the nervous system of the human and some animals. It is designed for students of medicine as well as the allied health professions.

Komáromy L: Brain Dissection, 5th ed. River Edge, NJ, Vanous, 1964.
Originally published as Dissection of the Brain, A Topographical and Technical Guide, Akadémiai Kiadó Budapest, Publishing House of the Hungarian Academy of Science.
This book contains a brief descriptive text and superb artist's drawings of the author's dissection technique. The complete dissection requires three brains. This book may be difficult to obtain.

LeMasurier HE: A simple method of staining macroscopic brain section, Arch Neurol Psychiat, **34**:1065–1067, 1935.

Matsui T, Hirano A: An Atlas of the Human Brain for Computerized Tomography. Tokyo, Igaku-Shoin, 1978.
This is the first among the several atlases that have appeared for CT scanning techniques. It is a monumental work containing labeled photographs and CT scans in many planes from 0° to 140° about the canthomeatal line.

Miller J: The Body in Question. London, Jonathan Cape Ltd., 1978.
An excellent book by a very articulate man. It is the author's commentary from the medical television series that bears the same title.

Miller RA, Burack E: Atlas of the Central Nervous System in Man, 3rd ed. Baltimore, Williams & Wilkins, 1982.

Mulligan JH: A method of staining the brain for macroscopic study, J Anat, **65**:468–472, 1931.

Nieuwenhuys R, Voogd J, van Huijzen C: The Human Central Nervous System: A Synopsis and Atlas. New York, Springer Publishing Company, 1978.
This book is beautifully illustrated with black and white artist's drawings and line diagrams that demonstrate both the structure of the brain and functional neuroanatomic circuitry.

Nomina Anatomica, 4th ed., New York, Excerpta Medica, 1977.

Roberts M, Hanaway J: Atlas of the Human Brain in Section. Philadelphia, Lea & Febiger, 1970.
This book is composed solely of photographs of surface-stained slices of the brain taken in the three basic neuroanatomic planes—coronal, parasagittal, and horizontal.

Romanes GL: Cunningham's Manual of Practical Anatomy, Vol. 3, Head and Neck and Brain, 14th ed. New York, Oxford University Press, 1978.

Sarnat HB, Netsky MG: Evolution of the Nervous System. New York, Oxford University Press, 1974.
A thought-provoking book on the evolutionary developments that probably determined in large measure the shape and structure of the human brain.

Snell RS: Clinical Neuroanatomy for Medical Students. Boston, Little, Brown and Company, 1980.
This is a textbook of neuroanatomy by a prolific writer who has written several other books on anatomical subjects. The book is well illustrated and has a section at the end of each chapter on clinical problems in neurology.

Watson C: Basic Human Neuroanatomy: An Introductory Atlas, 3rd ed. Boston, Little, Brown and Company, 1985.
This book contains summaries in note form of the major neuroanatomic pathways, photographs of the exterior of the brain, labeled brain slices, and histological sections through the brain stem.

Williams PL, Warwick R: Functional Neuroanatomy of Man. Philadelphia, WB Saunders Company, 1975.
This is an older but classical textbook in neuroanatomy that has been extracted from the larger Gray's Anatomy. Besides a definitive text and voluminous references, it contains many color photographs illustrating the structure of the brain.

Zuleger S, Straubesand J: Atlas of the Central Nervous System in Sectional Planes. Baltimore, Urban & Schwarzenberg, 1977.
As the title implies, this book contains artist's drawings of histological sections in the three basic neuroanatomic planes through the brain and transverse sections through the spinal cord.

The following books are no longer available in print but may be found in some libraries:

Aitken JT, Sholl DA, Webster KE, Young JZ: A Manual of Human Anatomy: Central Nervous system, Vol. V, 2nd ed. London, E & S Livingston Ltd., 1967.

Hewitt W: The Gross Anatomy of the Human Brain: A Manual of Dissection. London, Pitman Medical Publishing, 1967.
This book contains detailed instructions for the dissection of the brain in the neuroanatomy laboratory, but the illustrations are highly stylized drawings that do not represent what the student will observe in his own dissection.

Skinner HA: The Origin of Medical Terms, 2nd ed. Baltimore, Williams & Wilkins Company, 1961.
It is unfortunate that this book is out of print, for it is a scholarly work in which the author provides historical derivation for many of the gross neuroanatomic terms used in modern texts.

Index

Entries in boldface refer to illustrations. Entries followed by the letter "t" refer to tables.